SO GOD MADE RANGERS

T. SHANE PETTY

Copyright © 2023 by T. Shane Petty

All rights reserved.

DEDICATION

This book is dedicated to the appreciation of all rangers in the world but of course it goes without saying, especially for the Tennessee state park ranges I led and worked side by side on so many emergencies! The citizens of Tennessee owe a great debt of gratitude to these special men and women for their dedicated service 24-7-365.

This book is especially dedicated to my former Chief ranger who hired me as one of his assistants and pushed me in the direction of leadership and also to Park Manager Jim Hall. Jim worked his entire career of 44 years at Fall Creek Falls where he and I became good friends since we worked so many emergency calls together. In later years as his health was failing, he was always a phone call away to lend a helpful ear to my searches and how to approach them to be solved. He became a great mentor to me and asked only one thing, that I never make a trip to Fall Creek and not come see him!

He asked me to speak at his funeral as he was battling cancer and one thing that always stuck out to me when he said, "I don't mind dying but I just don't want to miss any emergencies"!

Well done, thy good and faithful servant""

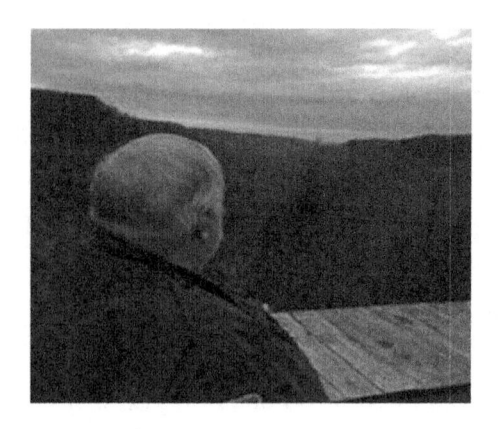

TABLE OF CONTENTS

In Memory 1
Special Thanks 3
Prologue for Shane 5
A Little Roman in The Smokies 7
In the Arms of an Angel 13
The Hanging Man Train Wreck 27
The Search for the Poison Mouthwash 29
The Missing Kayaker Mark and Scott's First Find 31
The Lost Tuber 35
The last time I saw Geoff Hood 39
Cumberland Trail North Chick Lost Couple 43
Duck River Canoeing Accident 47
Rock Island Miracle 49
Tennessee Highway Patrol Aviation 51
The Great Smokies Relationship 53
The Birth of the Green Air Splint 57
South Cumberland Carry Out 63
South Cumberland Hypothermia 67
Tri Corner Knob Hypothermic Hoist 71
Snagging a Trooper 75
Shelly Mook and Holy Bobo Searches 81
Searching for Fran 85
A Search at Andrews Knob 89

Sad Wrecks on the Highway 93
Rock Island Body Float Recovery 95
Radnor Lake Emergencies 99
Positive Identification..101
Plane Crash in the Smokies... 103
Plane Crash at Fall Creek Falls 107
Another THP Pilot Hero Ryan Quinn 111
Pickett Park Pup Search 115
Our Worse Rescue Cummins Falls Flood.......................117
Our First Accident Investigation 125
My Toughest Day.. 129
My First Rescue...131
Montgomery Bell Lake Find 133
Miracle in the Mountains.. 135
Harrison Bay Widow Maker..143
Greeter Falls Missing Person 145
Fort Loudoun State of Emergency 147
Fall Creek Tragedy...151
Fall Creek Falls Ghost 153
Fall Creek Falls 159
Fall Creek Falls Drowning... 163
Fall Creek Falls Campout Carryout 167
Drowning's on Duck River..173
July 4th Double Drowning...175
Diabetic Drowning Tailgate Drop 177
Derek Leuking Search in the Great Smokie Mountains ...179
Dickson County Vehicular Homicide 181
Cummins Falls Double Drowning................................... 187
Cumberland Trail North Chick Lost Couple 193

Burgess Falls High Angle Rescue	197
Burgess Falls Goat Man	201
Brad Lund	203
Brad Lavies, the Search that Changed My Life	209
Atlanta, I'm Coming to You Some Sweet Day	212
Arrow Suicide	215
A Nightmare at Standing Stone	217
My Last Search as Chief (And it was our biggest)	219
About the Author	241

INTRODUCTION

All my life I have been fascinated with the idea of a park ranger. A person who protected the people and resources of our wild areas! I was one of those fortunate ones who spent a career and a life doing such things, but I wanted to appreciate and applaud all rangers not only in Tennessee but all over the world!

Rangers are the most overlooked in most government entities and wear too many hats to count. They work daily to prevent emergencies, but it is always on our mind!

They spend their lives working when everyone else plays in the out of doors and when tragedy strikes, they are trained and prepared for all emergencies!

As you read this book, I hope you have a greater respect for rangers as they deal with too many tragic accidents and fatalities but please also keep in mind the families who lost a loved one due to one of these tragedies.

This book is a small snapshot of searches, rescues, and various emergencies that I worked alongside of my Tennessee state park rangers and after you read this book you will understand why I chose the title---*"So God Made Rangers"*

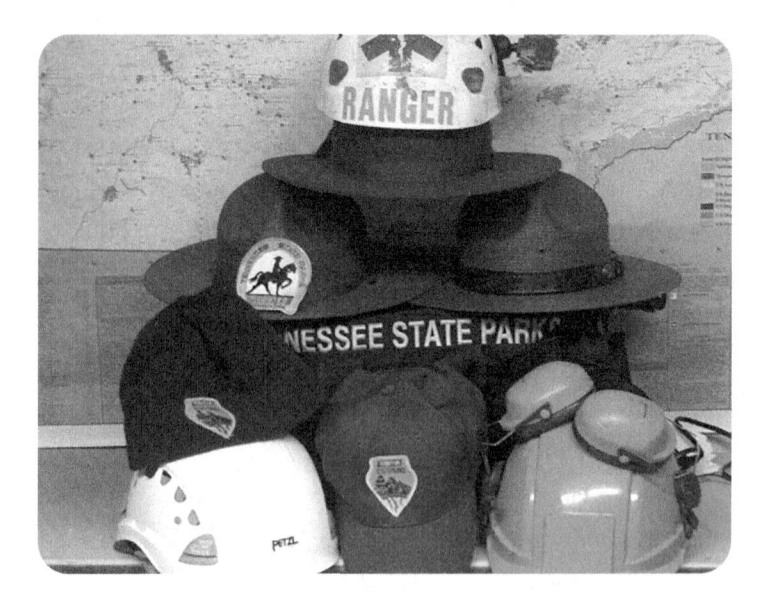

FORWARD

When it comes to search and rescues in Tennessee, the first name I think of is Chief Shane Petty. I was blessed enough to grow up in a Tennessee State Park due to my father being a Park Ranger. This gave me the good fortunes of meeting Chief Petty at a young age. Although most kids probably did not get the opportunity to go on search and rescues from a single digit age upwards, I did. Many of those rescues Chief Petty was leading the way. I could tell stories for days about the different rescues I went on with Chief Petty leading the charge, but instead I will just tell you many were successful rescues and some were not. However, that was just due to the circumstances and the severity of some of those rescues. Chief Petty was the type of man who repeatedly checked on the patients for those successful ones and the families for those that did not go well.

After finishing law school, I still saw Chief Petty routinely as he had me assist with new Park Rangers for the State. Chief Petty was constantly attempting to share his knowledge with those that came after him. This also gave me a great opportunity to see Chief Petty do different types of searches. Throughout his law enforcement career, he would search for fugitives using his blood hounds. At times, this also included searching for missing people and/or burial sites. As a former prosecutor and now a Judge, I have seen Chief Petty do nearly every type of search. If someone is looking for the foremost authority on searches and/or rescues, look no further than Chief Shane Petty.

M. Caleb Bayless

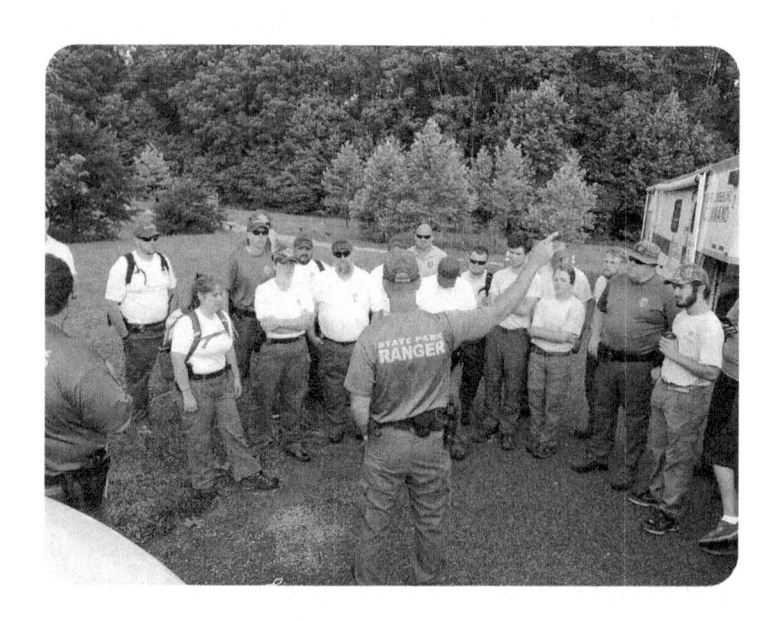

IN MEMORY

August 23, 2022, is a day many of us will never forget. Tennessee lost a dedicated law enforcement in Sgt. Lee Russell with Tennessee Highway Patrol aviation division and a hero to the citizens of Tennessee as he had already in his early career solved many cases with his helicopter and performed several rescues. His co-pilot that day was Detective Matt Blansett of Marion County and tragically this date they were killed in a helicopter crash on Aetna mountain in Marion County Tennessee.

Lee had the heart of a servant and a boyish grin that made everyone he met love him but I got to know him first with several helicopter rescues in the state but also he became my wing man on several cases I was working on the ground with my k-9 pursuing a fleeing felon. In my last K-9 case (Dickson County Homicide), Lee was once again my wing man as I tracked a suspect through the woods of Montgomery Bell state park. My k-9 Swabe trailed to the suspect and without any back up I requested Lee to land by my truck and enter the woods to cover the suspect while I searched him.

Lee was an officers officer giving his all to the profession! Lee went on to help me teach rangers and basic police officers when I taught at the police academy on manhunts! All of our hearts have an empty space in the loss of our friend who left behind his mom and dad, brother, wife and two small children.

All proceeds from this book will go to a scholarship fund for his two children.

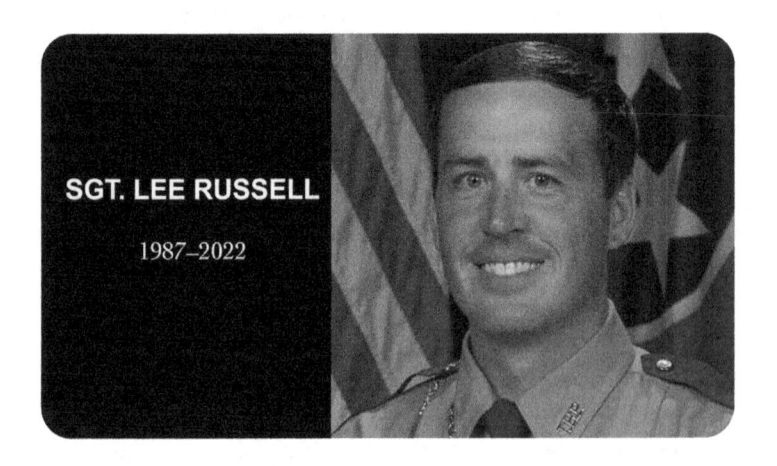

SGT. LEE RUSSELL

1987–2022

SPECIAL THANKS

Thank you to Arlyn Miller and my mom for proofreading and correcting, your time is greatly appreciated!

PROLOGUE FOR SHANE

It had been 24 years since I spoke to either of the two park rangers that came into view through the woods after I had been lost for 4 days in the Smokey Mountains. As we spoke on the phone and shared each of our perspectives of that event and our endeavors since, a flood of memories filled my head. Then came the chilling realization of how easily the search for 10 year old me could have had a different outcome. It's surreal to consider the choices of a naive and adventurous 10 year old could have resulted in death... my sister being raised as an only child, never seeing the pride on my parents face as I graduate college, neither the opportunity to serve in the US Army through two deployments, nor simply to take my nephew camping and fishing.

For years it was one of those events that I put in the back of my mind as I carried on with life. After I hung up the phone I pondered, "How lucky am I?!" Lucky that there's people that are not just willing, but capable and trained to search and rescue young dumb kids that go off trail. Shane Petty is one those of special people that make this world - and this country - a better place. If it wasn't for him and those that worked beside him that day it only was a matter of time before dehydration or hypothermia took a hold of me for the worst. I made a bad decision to go off trail, followed by both good and bad decisions on my part after I found myself lost. I was honored when Shane told me that those events in the summer of 1994 helped contribute to his involvement in and promotion of The Hug a Tree initiative. A program that shares with children the knowledge that could make the difference if they ever find themselves lost.

I still love the outdoors as much I did before that eventful summer, perhaps more. I now live in Alaska and camp over 30 days year... with proper navigation equipment and wilderness medicine training of course. If it wasn't for men like Shane Petty that answer the call of their communities I would not be sharing these words with you today.

As a survivor, my advice to those in trouble is "believe you will succeed. Where there's a will there's a way. Never give up."

And to those responders that answer the call "follow - and follow through - on your instincts and passions." The rest of us need you".

Phillip Roman—12/1/2018

A LITTLE ROMAN IN THE SMOKIES

In 1994 there were circumstances that would change and shape my life and career forever. I led a group of rangers from Tennessee to the Great Smokey Mountains National Park to assist in looking for a 10-year-old boy who had been missing for 3 days after being separated from his family.

Phillip Roman had traveled to Gatlinburg for a summer vacation at Dollywood, when the family decided to make a side trip to the national park and their trek to them to the parking lot of Clingman's Dome. Even though Phillip has always enjoyed and loved the outdoors he was not especially happy with this trip to the wilderness solely on the issue of not going to the park. As the family took in the sites from the observation tower, young Phillip decided he would take off alone back to the parking lot alone, however, the adventurous young boy decided to take a short cut through the woods to the parking lot.

As the family found themselves back at the parking lot, they discovered Phillip was not there. A quick search began by his dad and soon rangers from the national park were on the hunt for the 10-year-old. The Chief ranger for TSP at the time was Ed Schoenberger, and he was contacted by officials from the Tennessee Emergency Management Agency that the GSMNP rangers had requested assistance from us in the search for Phillip, who had been missing for two days. Unfortunately, Ed had just had eye surgery and could not make the trip, so he handed down the reins to me being one of the assistant chief rangers.

I spoke to Bob Swabe, who was an area coordinator for TEMA east which included the national park. Bob and Richard Taylor were the driving force in implementing the search management courses in Tennessee taking by thousands of police, fire, rescue squads, and rangers, including myself. During these courses, Bob knew I had a special interest in the search world, especially after the Brad Lavies search a year before but Bob knew there was something about me, he apparently liked.

I mustered up a team and we met at the park visitors center early in the morning and began a long day of searching but at the end of the day we did not find Phillip, however that evening Bob pulled me aside after the rangers gave us a debriefing and plans for the next day.

Bob told me that ranger's Pat Patton and staff tracker Dwight Carter had found tracks of Phillips docker shoes when he had stepped over a log. The sole of Brads shoes were a design of dozens of triangles and the ranges had found 4 of those small triangles, a virtual "needle in the haystack."

Bob had enough information from the NPS rangers that they really believed they were close to finding the young lost child. Bob told me he arranged it for me and another ranger (who was the other assistant chief), Bill Troop to a NPS team. The next morning, we headed out on the hike towards Clingman's Dome and then to the spur towards the

Appalachian Trail. After hiking for a bit, we took a turn down into a deep gorge towards the area the rangers had discovered the track. This was a very steep and treacherous hike, and it took us until almost noon to reach the area to search, so we stopped and took a quick lunch break and then headed out to search for Phillip. It wasn't but a few minutes we heard a voice yelling to us and as we hustled over the rise there was young Phillip, with a large smile on his face!

After medics from the park service checked him out, we shared a small bit of food and water to him and then the second most moving thing I have witnessed during a search happened. Our lead ranger radioed to the ranger's stationed at the parking lot to have Phillips' mom and dad be present with them close to the radio, then Phillip was allowed to make a statement on the radio that he was okay, and they would see him very soon at the parking lot.

Finally, it was time to bring Phillip back to his awaiting family, but it was going to be a tough climb out of that drainage! Phillip (who had been missing for 5 days) was weak and had sustained a leg injury, so we all took turns carrying Phillip on our backs as we headed straight up. If you have ever hiked to Clingmans Dome you know how deep the gorges seem but I will be the first to tell you even as a fit ranger of the age of 29 the elevation changed was extremely arduous. As we took turns carrying Phillip out on our backs you can understand that it would not take long to "tag out" with a team member to take Phillip for a few feet.

As we made the climb higher and higher the need to take breaks were often and we were exhausted from the searching as well as taking turns with Phillip but even though we were so tired everyone wanted him on their backs again, if only for a few feet. Once we were back on the AT spur Phillip was able to walk on his own back to the area where ranger's and his family were waiting. As we arrived Phillips dad ran to give him a big hug and then thank us but at that moment when we handed him to his mom, and I locked eyes with her as she hugged her baby boy and she uttered "thank you"!

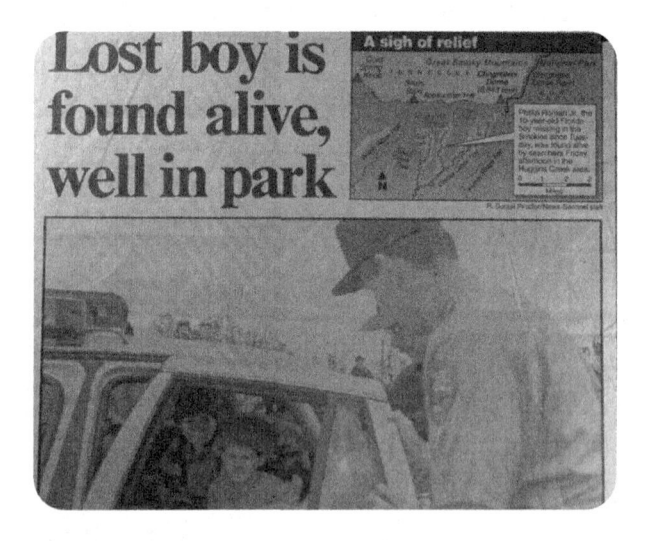

Lost boy is found alive, well in park

A sigh of relief

I had to walk away from the celebration due to the fact I was overcome with the emotions of the reunion, and I began to cry uncontrollably! This didn't seem a very macho thing for a ranger to do at this happy occasion, but it was the idea we saved the young boy, and I didn't have to see another mom heartbroken! Of course, this go without saying, this was the most moving thing I have ever witnessed and experienced!

In 2018 I began a search to find this little boy named Phillip. He no longer lived in Cape Corral Florida, and it seemed with all of my investigation ability and assets I was going to find him, until his sister replied to one of my dozens of social media post. I was able to begin a text dialogue with Phillip which eventually led to our meeting at the Tennessee/Georgia state line when he was visiting his dad. After our meeting and discussing several stories about that day, then we left and went on with our lives. A few days later sent me the following prologue of his account unsolicited.

IN THE ARMS OF AN ANGEL

The date was September 6, 1997, and the beginning of another mountaineer folk festival at Fall Creek Falls state park. I had been coming to Fall Creek for several years as a horse-mounted ranger to lend a hand to the staff during one of the busiest days in state parks! I had spent much of the day before welcoming school kids who were attending the festival and several visitors and campers stirring as vendors were still setting up shop. At some time that day a young man with a group had made visual contact with me and my horse and his thoughts came across to approach the horse for a friendly pet to amuse his friends, however, our paths would not cross until later that day.

As Saturday began, as with every folk festival I dashed to purchase the fresh chocolate and peach pies before they were gone! I completed grooming my horse "Velvet Elvis" and readied him for a long day in the saddle to greet the crowds as we had done so many times before not knowing the horrific tragedy that would happen later in the day!

Somewhere around midday, a call came over the radio that a girl had fallen and broken her leg at the bottom of the "cable trail" at the base of Cane creek falls. Ranger Dennis Bayless took the initial response to the call while the rest of us worked for the crowd at the festival until Dennis called on the radio that he could not find the injured lady. A medical call is a common occurrence, especially in this area but I remember thinking, " I am on a horse, what could I do, but for some reason, I decided to load the horse in the trailer and respond to assist my fellow ranger. When I arrived at the Nature center Dennis still had no contact with the girl and was going to head down the creek in search of her. The next actions I took were nowhere in the ranger manual and not taught in any rescue class but just on a whim and potential hypothesis of what may lie ahead or if could it be God calling me to help.

About a month before this day, I had decided to enroll in EMT school at Columbia state community college believing I needed to be a better medical responder for the visitors of Tennessee state parks even though I had met the minimum qualifications.

So, today I unloaded my mount, swung my medial bag on my back, and secured a 150-foot rope and my rappelling harness onto the saddle, an action I had never done before in any training scenario nor repeated since! Knowing I could never go down the "cable trail" I decided to traverse the

Paw Paw trail that ran along the ridge above the cane creek drainage taking a peek over the hedge every few yards to see if I could spot the injured woman. As frustration was mounting and the thought crossed my mind the woman may be in a different area when I finally spotted two individuals below me in the creek. I quickly tied my horse to a sturdy tree, threw on my rappelling harness, secured my rope with a sturdy bowline knot, and off the edge of the cliff I descended to a scene that was hard to describe.

23-year-old Laurel Paulus and her brother David were celebrating her birthday at Fall Creek Falls that weekend with several other friends at a local private campground. Laurel being the free spirit adventurous young woman had her whole life ahead of her, so she planned on exploring as much of the parks as she could that weekend. Laurel and David set out on their own to explore the Cane Creek drainage and rock hopping and rock-climbing small ledges to experience the full rush of the park. As Laurel was climbing around a large rock it gave way in her arms and she fell approximately 10 feet to the base of the creek. The 300-pound boulder landed on Laurel's petite body and left her damaged beyond belief! The main trauma to Laurel's body was found at her right hip where it was pinched by the boulder completely shattering her hip and almost completely amputating her leg.

David Paulus witnessed the most tragic nightmare unfolding in front of him without any time or ability to stop the boulder from its deadly fate. As he reached Laurel his worst thought was confirmed that she was completely crushed by the massive boulder and her life was taking a turn toward the worse. As he inspected Laurel's lifeless body the nightmare became even worse as the creek, she fell into had already become a bright red from the massive loss of blood from her crumpled body. David knew that he had to get help, but he also knew he had to do something to stop the bleeding and stabilize Laurel's leg so, he took off all of his clothes to use as a pressure bandage, splint, and tourniquet hoping to keep her alive until he could return with help! Adorned with only his boxers and boots he ran the creek back to the cable trail area and notified a passing car with individuals headed to a company picnic at the park to go get the help he returned to Laurel hoping for the best but afraid she may have passed away! The 45-minute race to go get help had to have seemed like an eternity as well as the same 45 minutes to race back to her only to find her head slumped back in a lifeless posture. As he made his way back to her body, he was overwhelmed she had survived his trip.

As I neared the bottom of the cliff face, I was unsure of what I had stumbled onto as I first found David in his new hiking uniform and attempting to explain to me what had happened. As I ran to the young lady in the water I felt as if I was in a horror movie as she lay in a large pool of bright red water. Without giving much thought to BSI I entered the water to prepare my patient for a long carryout when I gently raised her body finding that her leg was approximately 95% amputated and barely hanging on by a small amount of tissue. As I attempted to keep my composure in front of David, I felt the stare of this young ladies' eyes looking at me to save her life so, I swallowed hard and began the hardest and longest day of all of our lives!

As I asked ranger Bayless for his advice as to the best route out of the creek, he stated we would have to carry her in a stokes basket which was being brought by his son Caleb to the scene. As I raised her body again out of the water to inspect the clothing bandage applied by her brother I knew we were in trouble as the blood would quickly shunt back to the open injuries and drain Laurel from life so. I decided to lower her back into the water to stop the blood flow but also could tell the tremendous pain was also relieved by the cold water. I knew the cold water was more than likely the only thing that was keeping her from bleeding out so I would slowly raise her body only high enough to work the stokes basket under her body and then lower it back down.

I would now decide my life to remove Laurel's fading limp body out of the water and begin packaging her in the basket for the long carry out of the gorge. One of the most knowledgeable rangers of the gorge area besides Dennis was Stuart Carroll who had made his way to the scene with several other employees and volunteers. I have stuffed almost every piece of gauze bandaging into Laurel's wounds to slow the bleeding as we can on the long and arduous trek out. For some reason, I felt so connected to this young patient and I, like everyone, wanted her to make it out alive but we just had a bad feeling!

If you have never been in the drainage of cane creek it is lined with extremely large boulders 4-8 feet tall in some places making walking almost impossible without hopping from rock to rock. Other obstacles that would present a challenge were large pine and spruce trees that would create certain roadblocks causing us to go over or under with the basket.

It takes 40 good strong individuals to carry a Stokes basket for some time but when you add the terrain, we needed hundreds!

Someone at some point had recruited a group of people who were having a company picnic at the shelter close to the nature center to assist with carry out along with local rescue agencies from Piney. As we continued the carryout several had become seriously concerned with the amount of blood our patient was losing despite me holding as tight as I could to the femoral artery. Even though we in the medical field are taught to avoid all body fluids at any cost, this day found all of us on the basket covered in blood due to the shifting of the basket and the patient to get around the obstacles.

As we were getting closer to the falls and road, we knew we still had several issues to deal with that would determine if our patient would live. I radioed park manager Jim Hall to get a helicopter in route from Erlanger Hospital in Chattanooga when to my frustration one of the medical personnel on top with Jim said he was the only person who could make that call but not only after his inspection of the injured party. There are only a few times in my career that I became angry during an emergency, but I knew we were on the edge of death with Laurel, so I informed Jim that as the Chief of law enforcement I had the highest authority on the park and to get the helicopter ready. I also demanded that the paramedics meet us at the bottom of the cable trail to attempt an IV to get some fluids in her to keep her heart and major organs alive.

At one point we had to take a break to have fresh volunteers tend the basket so I attempted to check the vitals on our patient when I lost all hope when I could not find a heartbeat nor read any blood pressure. As I was about to tell our group I was afraid she has died, this young grey-pale girl looked at me and smiled and said, "Did I tell you it was my birthday?" As we once again began our journey, for some reason I cannot explain I began to sing "Happy birthday" to our patient! I guess to lighten the mood or to reassure her that all was going to be okay, but I knew time was not on our side!

As we were approaching the "cable trail" which is the long climb out of the gorge I was relieved when I heard Ray Cutcher was setting up a haul system and had dozens of volunteers to line the trail to pass the patient up. Ray, just like Stuart is the best of the best when it comes to rescues as he has organized hundreds if not thousands in his career as a ranger. We all knew even with the many volunteers lining the trail our patient would probably bleed out during the ascent due to the steep incline. I remember Ray was concerned with trying to keep her body horizontal for the climb to the top but there was just no time, we had to get her to the top!

We decided we would pass her off to the mass of people who now lined the trail but for some reason, I refused to leave her! From the first time I saw her mangled body, I was determined not to leave her side since she told me "Please don't let me die", so I mustered the last amount of energy I had with a large boost of adrenaline and off we went up the cable trail! Unfortunately, our prediction became real when we began the accent and blood began pouring out of her body once again all over us and we made the decision to stop halfway up the cable trail when we met the paramedics who attempted to begin an IV on her. I will never forget the look on the same medic's face when he saw how lifeless and the severity of her injuries he almost became passed out! After several attempts they could not get a line anywhere they attempted since her veins all became limp from no pressure and blood inside of them!

We decided to get her to the top of the road and into the ambulance and onto the waiting helicopter. As I made my way to Jim who had orchestrated all of the top commands he asked if she made it, I uttered "She somehow held on, but I don't believe she will make it to the hospital." We began our debriefing in the parking lot with each other on how we felt it went, what we did right, and what we wished we had done differently. As we finally came to the realization, we did all we could, and the cards were just stacked against us we decided it was time to return to the festival and try to resume back to normal life as a ranger.

Before we could make the next move, I will never forget the question from our group Caleb Bayless asking, "Shane, where is your horse?" At that moment I began to lose my mind thinking; was my horse still tied to the tree, had he got lost and fallen off the edge of the cliff, or a hundred things that may have happened to my faithful partner? My love for my horse was just as deep as it was for my family so I asked Caleb to rush down the "Paw Paw" trail to see if he could find him. As Caleb departed, he asked me "Chief if I find him can ride him back?" After a quick ponder I said NO! After a long wait, he returned with my steed, and we loaded him in the trailer and we both decided it was time to call it a day!

I awoke early that Sunday morning just like all of the rangers at Fall Creek to begin another busy last day of the festival. As we began our ritual of buying up the fried pies before they were gone, I attempted to mount my horse when I found my legs were so tight and sore, I had to use a picnic table! After a few hours, I ran into Jim and we discussed the day we had before and both wondered, "You think she made it?" Jim contacted Ellen Geesling who worked with EMS at Erlanger Hospital, and she told us "She is alive!"

After the festival was over, I dreaded the long drive back home, but something told me to go to the hospital and lay eyes on this miracle! Security was not thrilled to make accommodations for the horse, but they granted me first-class parking and helped me make it to intensive care. After several requests to make it in a doctor came out to see me and asked if I was on the rescue. After confirmation, he told me we pulled off one of the most impressive things he had ever seen by keeping a person alive with the most serious injury he has ever encountered. He also told us she had about 15 minutes to live when she arrived at the hospital due to the fact, they put 11 liters of blood into her system.

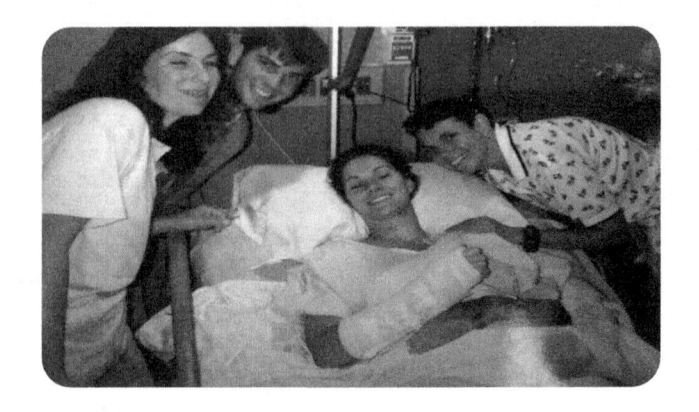

As he took me into the ICU, he introduced me to Jim Paulus (Laurel's dad) and he then took me to Laurel's bedside I stated that "I don't think this is the same girl", something about her skin tone wasn't right. The doctor said she looked grey and ashen when you saw her because she had bled almost to death but that "we saved her life, pure and simple!" I don't think I have ever seen so many tubes. As I left the hospital I felt as if I were on cloud nine knowing that I was part of a miracle and beaming knowing "she made it"!

For many years to come, I took Laurel with me in many aspects of my life. My job is to teach and facilitate rope rescue training as well as medical training for all Tennessee park rangers. This incident also spurred me to take over the medical training for the Tennessee Law Enforcement Academy for every police officer in the basic police school from 1996 still today! Laurel's story also pushed me to hold several blood drives during our ranger in services raising hundreds of pints of blood always in her honor knowing blood is what saved her life!

For many years my mind would wonder about Laurel and whether was she still alive, did she ever walk again, did graduated college, did she have a family, and if she even remembered that day. Over the past year after writing a book on my k-9 experiences, I decided I would make it my duty to find this girl that was always in the back of my brain driving me to help others! I remembered that a good friend and former ranger Alan Wasik's family had gone to church with the Paulus family in Dickson. I made my way to Strawberry Plains and found Alan and his wife Judy and spent a great evening with them discussing old times and rescues! I asked Alan if he could reach out to his mom and try to get a phone number for Mr. Paulus.

In December 2019 I was able to finally talk to Jim Paulus (Laurel's dad) and he immediately remembered me coming to the hospital to visit Laurel. We spoke for a long time that night but when he told me Laurel had been living in Colorado for the past twenty years my heart sank a little knowing I may never get to see her again but at that moment he changed my life. He told me Laurel had moved back to Tennessee and was living in Nashville and he gave me her contact information.

It took me several days to muster the words to open a conversation and gain the confidence to contact her in hopes she would be willing to talk to me. We traded messages for a few days and finally made an appointment to meet in Brentwood which made me happy but also very nervous after 22 years! As I sat in the restaurant I wondered "Would I even recognize her", "Would she remember me", would she be in a wheelchair", and "Would we have anything to talk about"?

Being in uniform I aimlessly walked around the restaurant waiting for her to flag me down but no Laurel! I took a booth where I could see the door and anxiously watched every person enter the room trying to picture her face from so many years ago! All of a sudden there she was, I knew that face as it was yesterday, and I met her halfway noticing only a small limp and we gave each other a hug knowing we both needed that re-connection after so many years!

We began our conversation with Laurel telling me the numerous surgeries she has undergone with hundreds of staples, metal plates, and hip replacements! We then dove into our accounts of the day and compare notes of who, what, when, and where! It was obvious she had traveled down the road of remembering the day, but I was struggling to go back to that day. Most everything came back to us but the most important thing that touched me that stopped me in my tracks is when Laurel asked, "Do you remember singing happy birthday to me". I immediately replied, "Why would I have sung to her during this terrible time", when it hit me that I could hear myself walking with the basket and singing to her after she kept telling me it was "MY BIRTHDAY"! I guess I gave in to her request to pass the time but down deep I knew this might be the last time she ever heard this song on this earth, and it was my duty to fulfill her last wish!

After we left that day, I could not stop smiling just as I had done that day leaving the hospital but as I entered my vehicle, I began to uncontrollably cry sitting in the parking lot which lasted for a long time on the way home! I guess the emotion of the day and re-encountering the event pushed my emotions but also knowing she made it in life and gave birth to two daughters! After a bit of driving even though I felt great about the day I felt as if she was gone again never to see or talk to her again, but I guess that is how life is!

After much thought, I realized Laurel's story needed to be heard and she and I should share our story. After much thought, I pushed the idea to her to speak at our park ranger in service in front of 244 officers. She was a little hesitant but was warming up to the idea when I felt like I had to give her some encouragement so without hesitation I told her "Don't forget you owe me for saving your life"! We had a good laugh and she agreed to take on the engagement, so our plan was in place. I have been involved in 30 years of service but never have I witnessed what Laurel brought to our ranks. I opened the door with the tragedy, and she brought the house down by letting us know "We were all chosen to do this job and we all had a destiny to be the protector of our park visitors"! She closed in service by stating, "She owed her life to many medical personnel, volunteers, but most importantly to park rangers"! All the rangers were speechless as me and had to wipe away tears from our eyes!

At the closing of the service, I remembered a question that ranger Mark Houston asked me the night before, "Chief, what was your best day in Tennessee state parks"? As I choked down the tears and struggled to find my voice I uttered to Mark and the room full of colleagues, "Laurel was my BEST DAY"!

THE HANGING MAN TRAIN WRECK

I was contacted one evening by the Marshall County Sheriff's Department to see if I could assist on River road where a train had just collided with a truck and they needed someone to get there and determine if the driver and passengers needed medical intervention.

I was home eating supper at the time when the call came to me and for some reason that day, I had parked in the front yard close to the porch, so I ran to the front door to make my response, however as I ran out the door I ran into a BIG problem!

As I threw the glass door open to make my exit the door swung back very quickly as I was about to descend the steps when the handle on the door hooked through my uniform shirt and created a hole in my shirt! Anyone who has ever worn a 100% polyester shirt, you are very aware of how rugged and durable the material can be. As I attempted to get to my vehicle, I was all of a sudden jerked violently back by the door handle that had penetrated my shirt! Also, it is very important to note at this point that the porch has a very small landing area which proved to be a significant issue when the door snatched me backward and off the porch!

I found myself dangling from the door handle hooked to my shirt and my feet would not reach the ground or the porch, so I was stuck in the air! I made several attempts to free myself by bouncing to rip the shirt, but the polyester would not let me go! After several attempts, I sat there just dangling from the door and trying to figure out my next course of action which was either rip the shirt or pull the door off the hinges but neither seemed to do the trick when my worst nightmare came across my mind!

As I hung there motionless, I could hear several sirens in the distance but I knew they would have to drive right by my house to get to the train wreck site and I knew I would never be able to outlive the humor that local first responders would get from me hanging myself during an emergency. The embarrassment that went through my body motivated me enough to finally rip the shirt and allow myself to drop to the ground.

I was able to respond to the train wreck (thankfully ahead of the sirens) and determined that my good friend Trey Lawrence was the driver of the vehicle he was unharmed but very lucky to be alive and now you know the real story that almost was!

THE SEARCH FOR THE POISON MOUTHWASH

I received a call from TEMA one Saturday morning and they transferred a frantic woman to me who was desperate to find her family, however, she was Asian, and I had a lot of trouble understanding her dialect. Apparently from what I could gather from our conversation her husband and son had gone camping and the mouthwash bottle they had taken with them was poison! To make matters worse she was almost hysterical so that added to the communication issue.

After trying to wrap my head around the idea this was a real situation, I began to ask her where they may have gone camping and she had no idea! The first question I had for; "Are they in Tennessee", the answer was yes but she was not sure if they were in a National or Tennessee state park. I then asked if they were camping in an R.V. or tent camping and we finally got it narrowed down to a tent. Unfortunately, this was the time before an electronic database so I could not run their name on our computer so I kept asking questions like which area of the state, but she had no idea.

I decided to see what type of recreation they may be doing and maybe this would lead me to their location. The lady on the phone finally told me they would be hiking (every park has a hiking trail) but I got enough information from her to narrow down more backcountry hiking and camping. I took her name and number and told her I would do my best, but in my head, I knew this was almost an impossible task.

I took a look at my state park map and just gambled on South Cumberland state park. I called the Stone Door Rangers station and interpretive specialist Randy Hedgepath answered the phone. I told him of the odd predicament and asked if he could check his camper registrations for the name and after several minutes of looking, I was floored when he said, "They came in last night"! I asked him to get to them as soon as possible to inform them of the poison mouthwash and call me back!

This was before cell phones in state parks but what seemed like forever Randy called me back within an hour to say he found the man and son and fortunately, they had not used the mouthwash! That was probably my quickest blind search ever, not bad for less than an hour!

THE MISSING KAYAKER
MARK AND SCOTT'S FIRST FIND

I was called back to the North Chick area of the Cumberland Trail when we received reports of an overdue kayaker. This case had a few bad starts, first, the water was about 9 feet above flood stage, secondly, the missing hiker did not tell anyone where he was going and entered the water by himself. My seasonal Mark Matzkiw and I loaded the mobile command center and rescue trailer and headed once again toward Chattanooga.

Cumberland Trail rangers Basham and Andy Wright had been on the search, but the swollen waters made it all but impossible to perform any type of water search. I had assembled a group of rangers from across the state to meet us there for the search which would be by foot. The initial information came in that the co-worker of the missing boater reported him missing when he didn't show up to work but we unfortunately had no one that could give us a boat color or description of his clothing and to make matters worse we had no good idea of where he put in his boat.

The North Chick drainage creek is wide but mostly shallow in many places but does have many deep holes when the area receives a large amount of water it makes for an attractive race track for kayakers but this day the water to dangerous even for the most experienced kayaker. This individual made the grave decision to go by himself and with the water level only an expert should attempt.

The only thing we had going for us was a break in the weather which allowed for the water to reseed a few feet so we could have a chance at spotting some type of clues. We had a crew of about 12 rangers and there was a group of local responders from Hamilton County STARS. After a planning session with rangers and manager Booby Fulcher, we began far upstream above his vehicle where we hypothesized the location he may have put in his boat.

Walking along the rocky bank is a very rough and slow process but we also had to add a large element of a risk assessment to our plan so that no one got hurt. The search was slow, but the rangers were doing their best with the hazardous slick and muddy rocks. At this point, we had the family on the scene so that always puts added pressure on you as a searcher but also the planner, and since I was the incident commander, I had a lot of pressure to find our boater.

It was getting up in the day and even though the search still had several hours left of daylight left it was time to put together a plan for the next day. Our concern was the amount of water and how fast it was flowing which could carry a body downstream for many miles making a search plan stretches to many days. My seasonal Mark Matzkiw was a seasonal searcher mainly because I had drug him along for many searches since so, I paired him up with Scott Ferguson from Cedars of Lebanon. The two were on the river right and very young and strong so they were like Billy goats combing the creek bank. They had worked across the Dayton highway where the creek makes a sharp turn close to the train track when they made the call for a "green air splint", which you know by now they had found our boater.

Our next steps are to confirm he is our missing person and also turn it over as an investigation to TWRA since it was a boating accident. I contacted my colleague Matt Majors once again to assist with that process. The next step was to notify the next of kin who was there on site. This is never an easy time, but it is the next step in recovery to allow the family to begin the grieving process. It is never easy at either party to tell a family their loved one has been found deceased but it is a job I do not wish on anyone. It tears at your heartstrings knowing the family will be changed forever.

After the investigation, we assisted in packaging the body which had been lodged at the base of a tree on a higher area of the bank which allowed us to find his body quicker since it was not in the main channel. We musted up at the command center where I conducted a debrief to make sure we learned from our experience and to make any changes to get better. We departed back to our areas of the state, but my job was not over, "the mission is not over until everyone returns home".

This is why God made a ranger!

THE LOST TUBER

The call came in as drowning at the North Chickamauga drainage area of the Cumberland Trail. These are the hardest calls because you just never know when it will be over! The Chattanooga area had seen a ton of rain and the normally small creek was swollen to dangerous levels when a group of people decided to float the water in tubes.

The party of 5 parked in the parking lot and headed upstream for a pretty good hike when they decided to get into the dangerous water. Two of the members turned over as soon as they touched the water, and the others flipped a few feet down from the launch. With the size of the roaring water, it is a miracle that all of them did not drown but one man did not surface.

Once the other individuals were able to drag themselves out of the water they began to run the creek bank in attempts to find their friend but those attempts were not successful and the outcome looked bad! One of them ran back to the car and called 911 and that initiated the C.T. rangers and local responders. Ranger Basham was coordinating the local responders and I began my job to respond to Chattanooga and muster state resources.

When I got to the park the parking lot was full of rescue trucks and personnel and there had been no success in finding the young man, so we were pretty sure we had a body recovery on our hands. The water was too high and dangerous for anyone to attempt any type of water search but we did have a few rangers who are experts in kayaks on the water. As the search continued with rangers and rescue responders walking the banks the only other resource, I could think of was to use Brad and his helicopter so he responded and flew at tree-top heights combing the creek.

I was at my truck and decided to do an old trick I learned from rescue responders at Fall Creek years ago by setting a fenced trap to catch the body. Stretch a fence across the creek and if the body floats down undetected or at night the fence will hold the body from going further downstream and expanding your search area. If you haven't been to the parking lot of the trailhead it is very small at best and designed for just a few dozen cars and as I was witnessing too many rescue, rangers, police, and fire responders I decided to get out of the lot before I was trapped in. Just as I pulled out onto the road a large fire engine pulled into the lot and I knew there was no room for that and I made a great decision.

I ran to the local TSC down the road to buy a fence and was returning downstream to set up the fence at the highway bridge when a call came over the radio that a neighbor downstream of the park spotted the body floating down the creek. Unfortunately, my thought came true in the parking lot and the engine was stuck being too big for the lot and no responders could get out of the parking lot to respond. I was only a few hundred feet away, so I drove to the end of the road at the neighborhood, threw on my PFD and grabbed a throw rope, and ran to the creek. I quickly spotted the body where it was held up for a second in a shallow spot of the creek so to make sure he didn't lose him again, I jumped in the water and grabbed him.

It was good to have the remains in my hand for the moment, but the other responders were still trapped and my only assistance was my good friend and EMA director Tony Reavley, who had not gotten to the parking lot yet. He and a few other firemen threw down a rope and we began to get out man for closure to the search so the family can begin the grieving process.

Even though the grieving can begin after a find you must also finish the investigation and it was a very sad finding to know the group stopped at a small drug store where they bought kid-type tubes. By the way, we quickly decided to make an arrangement at the local church on the highway for any further rescues, so we never get trapped again!

THE LAST TIME I SAW GEOFF HOOD

My first introduction to Geoff Hood was when we were both seasonals with Tennessee state parks. I was stationed at Cedars of Lebanon and Geoff got Henry Horton (of course that is where I wanted because it was close to home) but I was just happy to be a member of Tennessee state parks! I began to make so many new friends at our first training in service as so many new seasonal rangers, recreators, and interpreters but Geoff and I seemed to hit off immediately. We became friends in our short time together and decided we would touch base as much as we could since I would pass by Henry Horton on my way home.

As the summer went along, I would stop by as promised to see Geoff and we would talk about our programs, challenging visitors, and the future. We both had outdoor careers and lives planned and all seemed right! I remember it like it was yesterday the day I last saw Geoff. I had stopped by Horton, as usual, to get caught up, but Geoff was hard at work because I saw him as soon as I turned into the park driving a tractor and pulling several campers in a hay wagon. I followed him for a few seconds but stopped in the curve by the ranger houses and decided to turn around, not to bother him at work.

What I didn't realize two big things happened that day that would be with me for the next 35 years. The two ranger houses where I last saw Geoff both became my houses when I was hired as a ranger and later Chief ranger but the curve where I last saw Geoff haunted me still to this day. Every time I travel that route, which has been every day since my house and office were in this area, I can still picture Geoff on that old Long tractor.

Unfortunately, like many of us, we did not do a good job of keeping in touch and we grew apart after we returned to school. In the fall of 1990, I was completing my first complete year as a ranger at Henry Horton (where Geoff was stationed) and the word began to come in about one of the worse tragedies to ever happen on the Appalachian Trail on September 13th, a young man and woman had been murdered on the trail. Unfortunately, as more information flowed in it was discovered that the murdered couple was Geoff and his girlfriend Molly LaRue.

Molly and Geoff had begun the 2,180-mile trail hike earlier that year and like any through hikers they had met many other hikers along the way and made instant friends with everyone that their paths had crossed. The couple had stayed in a motel for hikers in Duncannon, Pennsylvania on September 11, where they had called their parents to meet them the next week at a half point to tell them some information (which both family members believed they were going to announce their engagement).

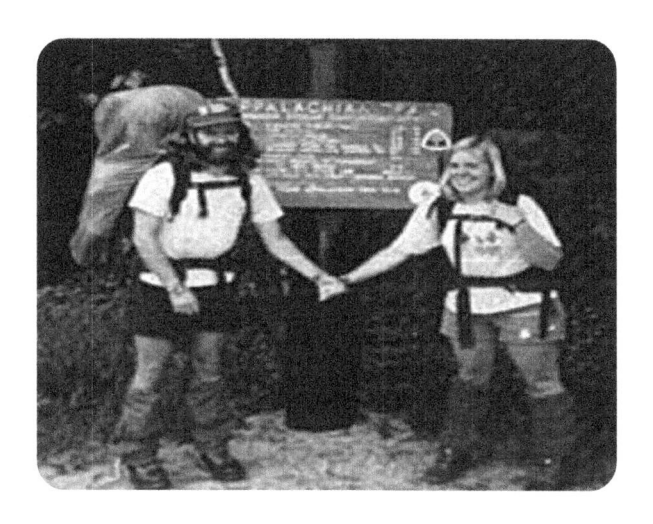

On the night of the 12[th,] they arrived back on the trail at the Thelma Marks shelter on top of Cove Mountain. Unfortunately, that night would be their last night on earth, sometime around 2:00 a.m. Paul David Crews entered the shelter and shot Geoff 3 times in the back and killed Molly with a knife. Crews had been on the lamb for several years suspected of a murder in Florida. He had spent time in West Virginia hiding with his brother when he decided to try to hide out on the trail.

Seven days later Crews was apprehended on the trail at Harpers Ferry, West Virginia wearing Geoff's boots and backpack. In 1991 he was sentenced to death, but later in 2006, the sentence was changed to two consecutive life sentences with no chance of parole.

Geoff has crossed my mind many times as I wondered how his life would have impacted so many others along with Molly. Many years later I discovered my daughter-in-law's mom Shelia had grown up with Geoff spending time at school and church functions. She was able for me to make contact with Geoff's mother, and we spent a morning in 2019 discussing Geoff's life I wanted her to know that Geoff's life is still remembered by many.

CUMBERLAND TRAIL NORTH CHICK LOST COUPLE

In early April of 2007 I received a call from ranger Daniel Basham of the Cumberland Trail that they had two teenagers that had gone hiking on the trail very near dark. They were not prepared hikers as they lived in a nearby neighborhood and were more out on a date away from parents. The parents had contacted ranger Basham and they did what the C.T. ranger did best most of their lives, hit the trail to find the lost!

After a long and exhaustive search of several miles of trail to the loop rangers couldn't locate the teens so, that is when I get the call. "Bash" gave me all of the details and with every search I look at the weather and age of the lost person and that determines our "search urgency"! It was early spring but the weather was seasonal warm and the teens were young and strong so we decided not to risk the safety of any other rescue personnel in the treacherous mountains. I decided since they went in there to as a couple, they would get a chance to hug all night!

I made a call to the emergency agency for my friend Brad Lund with THP to see if he could fly it the next morning but I had talked to him earlier in the day and knew he was scheduled to assist Maury county sheriff's department with their annual Mule Day but maybe he could give me a few hours. As I called the agency a supervisor told me the pilot was out of town and I became pretty furious and called him directly and in the best Brad Lund professionalism he said " I have to be in Columbia at 11:00 but I can give you a few hours.

Due to many incidents in this area Brad and I already had our own landing zone close to the park so I agreed to meet him at the LZ at 8:00 a.m. I arose early and drove to meet Brad and help the C.T. rangers with the day's search. This is a very steep and dangerous trail where one wrong step can lead to a severe injury so we were prepared for anything but very concerned since the kids were not found on the trail and did not return home. Brad landed in our designed bank parking lot landing zone and took off for the trail in search of our lost hikers.

The trail was still under construction and not yet connected to other areas of the trail but the trail is inside a 7000 acre natural area so we knew they could be lost deep in the wilderness. The trail climbs from the two entrances to the top of the gorge above the North Chickamaunga creek for several miles but eventually dropping back into the creek gorge. I am not positive of the altitude from the tree tops to the creek but it has got to be a few thousand feet in elevation so when Brad topped the trees he made no hesitation to drop down into the gorge almost giving me a heart attack but you cants see from that height so we began our search. Unfortunately the canopy is very dense in this area and this time of year adds many leaves so trying to spot them on the trail or off the trail would be almost impossible so, Brad decided our best bet would be to fly the creek drainage hoping they may have made it to the creek safely.

We had only flown the creek gorge for a few minutes we Brad said, " I got em"! They were apparently cold and huddled together as expected but fortunately the sun was helping to warm the rock so we were glad they were in good shape. Brad flew over them so we could get a thumbs up from them and then he asked if I had extra water in my bag and he lowered down to pitch the two bottles of water. I said "wouldn't be better for me to do it since you are flying"? In Brad Lund's cool demeanor, he said, "this aint my first rodeo, give me the water"!

We were able to relay the coordinates of the two kids to ranger Basham and Brad flew me back to the truck where we both made are way back to Columbia for Mule Day, of course he beat me by 4 hours!

DUCK RIVER CANOEING ACCIDENT

A call came one day that a canoer on the Duck river had fallen while out exploring a cave on the river. At that time the park was a canoe take out for a local canoe livery system and we had our share of injuries and emergencies associated with the recreation sport. A man was laying in the bottom of a canoe while other friends were rushing to get him to the take out. As I inspected the gentleman he was alert and talking to me but was lying in a large pool of blood in the canoe.

The gentleman had made a bad decision to get out of the canoe and attempt to hike up the step limestone slick rock face of a cave when he slipped and fell approximately 14 feet. He fell on the hard rock bank but during the fall he had apparently struck a sharp rock on the way down in the area of his neck and I became very concerned when I noticed the blood spurting from his neck which indicated a true emergency and he had more than likely punctured his femoral artery.

I immediately called for an ambulance and entered the canoe that was now on solid ground and began to apply a large pressure bandage on the large gapping hole in attempts to slow or hopefully stop the bleeding. The man never lost consciousness and seem to be in good spirits despite the injury. The ambulance got to the scene quickly and we loaded him in the vehicle and paramedics began to administer an I.V.

to help with the blood loss. I was glad to have the ambulance crew now stationed only a few miles from the park and hoped and believed we had got to him in time to save his life.

Later that evening the crew stopped by my house to inform me that the man had passed away while on his way to the hospital from apparent internal bleeding from the injury. It is very hard to process anytime you have a major accident but even harder when you lose a patient you worked so hard on to save their life!

ROCK ISLAND MIRACLE

After a long weekend searching for a drowning victim at Rock Island, I had returned back to retrieve our mobile command center and as I was about to pull out onto highway 70 I witnessed a van on the opposite side of the highway from me pull out onto the highway right in front of an 18 wheeler that was traveling approximately 65 MPH. The van that was full of young girls returning from a summer church camp and for some reason the driver either ran the stop sign or did not see the 18 wheeler and I witnessed the worst tragedy of my life!

As the collision began the van was struck right in the side and rolled over several times and each time it rolled over I would see a young girl thrown from the van onto the highway! As the 18 wheeler truck attempted to stop after the collision I was already on the phone with 911 and told them we needed several ambulances and possibly more than one helicopter due to the mechanism of injury and multiple victims. I had a bit of trouble getting the truck and command trailer parked in a safe place and then grabbed my medical kit and ran to the van very afraid of what I was about to see with my eyes.

I ran to the carnage on the ground of 11 young girls and began a triage of my victims from worse to those who had the best chance for survival but as I worked my way down the long line of victims each one would look at me with frightened eyes for help but one by one every girl would say my leg hurts or my arms hurts but unbelievable they were ALL conscious and seemed to have no outward life threatening injuries!

I began to clean wounds and bandage several road rash scrapes and bruises on every girl but also my attention turned to the possibility one or more of them may have a life threatening internal damage, so I began another systematic check from head to toe of each girl only finding more scares and contusions but no sign of internal bleeding! As I was about to deplete all bandages and gauze in my medical kit I heard that wonderful sound of sirens and EMS to assist. I ran to meet the arriving paramedics and gave them my report on injuries I had discovered and they too were astonished at the outcome! They did transport a few of the girls to the hospital for precaution but every girl turned out to be fine!

There was no doubt that God had put a hedge of protection around the van that saved those girls lives that day and reminded me the importance of my job as an EMT and to always be prepared!

TENNESSEE HIGHWAY PATROL AVIATION

Early in my career, I heard the name Mike Dover. Mike was a Vietnam veteran with two tours of duty and thousands of wartime hours in helicopters. He was very proactive in the '70s and 80's to take Tennessee aviation within the highway patrol to new heights. He was responsible for law enforcement air support for the state but also developed some of the first search and rescue plans as well as patient evacuation in rugged areas.

He trained many THP special operations tactical squad members but was instrumental in the Tennessee Mountain Rescue training within Tennessee state parks led by Bobby Harbin. Mike trained rangers how to package a patient in a Stokes basket for helicopter hoists out of areas such as Fall Creek Falls. He is credited with over 19,000 hours in the air. Mike and his son Tim Dover are great friends and retired Captains from THP who spent many hours helping Tennesseans in their time of need.

Dennis Kent is to say a character who was also a retired Lt. with the THP and was my first introduction to THP on the working level. He flew many flights over me looking for criminals but also worked with us continuing the Mountain Rescue. He was grateful to let me rappel out of the aircraft on many occasions and tag along on rescues. I worked with

Dennis several years during the Governors Marijuana Drug Task Force especially when he flew in a state park. I am thankful he let me fly with him on many occasions, but he also found plenty of marijuana at Fall Creek and he got his money out of us on the ground cutting it!

Thanks to these forward-thinking men for all you did for us in state parks!

THE GREAT SMOKIES RELATIONSHIP

Early in my career, I was part of a search team from Tennessee state parks under the direction of Chief Ranger Ed Schoenberger that was called to search for Brad Lavies which began my drive and desire to help those who were lost. Many of the stories you will find in their own story in this book.

A few searches ended in tragedy. That was the case of 13-year-old Brad Lavies, of Adamsville, Ala., who disappeared in 1993 while hiking to Rainbow Falls on Mount LeConte with family members. He was missing for six days before searchers found him dead in a creek at the base of a 100-foot cliff. ★ See story (Brad Lavies)

The next year I was handed the reins to be in charge of the team that would return to the mountains on the search for little Phillip Roman I was fortunate to be on the team that brought him out of the mountains and returned him to his mom and dad! ★ See (A Little Roman in the Smokies)

The next search was for Jennifer Dates who became separated from her hiking party on Rainbow Falls in bitter cold weather. One of the next searches I recall was for a missing hiker named Goherley who had a GPS unit that was running low on batteries which made it a challenge to find him due to the fact he kept moving. ★ See (Miracle in the Mountains)

Another search I headed up with the National park service turned into a search inside another in mid-March of 2012 when I took a search team to look for Joseph Leuking who had left behind all of his worldly possessions and disappeared into the smokies where he had abanded his car with a note in it stating "don't come looking for me. I took several rangers which included Jacob Ingram and Mark Matzkiw into an area from New Found Gap deep into the woods where we got caught in a terrible downpour but more importantly I told Jacob to better secure the GPS unit on his pack that I had given him but not heeding to my call he later had to tell me he lost the unit in a drainage. I immediately sent him back into the drainage in an attempt to find the unit but he returned with no luck and I will always remind him of that day and his not listening to his Chief! * See (Derek Leuking Search in The Smokies).

Oddly enough the park actually had a report of another missing person which was a probable suicide closer to the spur so Park manager Eric Hughey led a search team in the area but they could not find anyone, however a few years later the body of a man they were looking for was found in a very deep and thick Laurel thicket.

I was involved with several rescue/recoveries with the Tennessee Highway patrol aviation team ut our most notable was the recovery of a hiker who died from hypothermia on the A.T. (see Tri Corners Knob).

There were several other cases we worked on such as the Gourley search as well as Jenny Bennett who was a popular "off trail" hiker" who became missing in the park. I sent a group of rangers to assist in the case but her body was found just as they arrived, so the TSP rangers assisted the NPS rangers in the long carry out of her body.

In 2017 NPS officials requested us to assist them on a missing teenager who went missing in the park and had not been seen for several days. Rangers had several search teams looking for the teen but later it was discovered he was very mobile and continuously moving making it very hard to pin point his location. TSP rangers were being transported in by boat when he was spotted by a bass fisherman after 11 days. He was checked out at the hospital in great shape!

In 2018 I was requested to bring a team to the Smokies to aide in the search for Susan Clements who became lost after hiking the Forney Ridge trail in attempt to make it back to the Clingmans Dome parking lot. Several TSP rangers spent several days searching areas adjacent to Andrews Bald. Unfortunately, I, was suffering from bone spurs and awaiting surgery but I caught a ride with THP to assist from the air. The weather had visibility at a terrible and poor distance, but we searched as well as we could in the thick cloud cover at the high elevation. Her body was later found by a team of Tennessee troopers in the Huggins creek drainage where it was determined she died of hypothermia, close to the same area we found Phillip Roman years before.

THE BIRTH OF THE GREEN AIR SPLINT

The first major search I was involved with was in! 998 at Fall Creek Falls which unfortunately turned into a 13-day body recovery. The park manager Jim Hall called just to let me know he had it covered but I kind of begged and forced my way into the search and began the drive to the plateau expecting it to be a long week but never expecting a long two weeks! Jim and I had only had a few cordial meetings and paths crossing and of course, I was the new rookie who had not been tested so Jim was a bit apprehensive about me sharing the search command but after this search, we both began an admiration and appreciation for each other as well as a 20-year close friendship.

As with most all searches my job was to assist in command but also work logistics for state park resources and other state assets to help bring home the missing. A young man who was rock climbing decided to scale the low head dam at the George Hole by walking across its swollen spillway when his feet were apparently swept out from under him, and he was swept downstream! Another man that was with him ran down the creek to rescue his friend and almost had him out of the water when the current proved too strong and took his friend from his grasp. A few hundred yards downstream a family who was crossing the bridge witnessed the lifeless-looking body floating face down across the rapids towards the cascades which proved in the search arena that there was a point last seen and certainly a real search that would prove to be the longest in Tennessee state parks history.

Unfortunately, Fall Creek rangers have had a great deal of search experience in searches and their fair share of body recoveries, so Jim had his cadre of ranges and employees executing all aspects of a search but when I arrived is became aware more than likely this would be a body recovery. Ranger Ray Cutcher headed up a team of searchers in attempts to use pike poles to search rocks and strainers below the point last seen (PLS) where a body may become trapped. Interpretive Specialist Stuart Carroll was using teams to scour the cascades behind the nature center, but our main concern was did the body make it to the Cane Creek waterfall and either be at the bottom or even worse swept further downstream! Certainly the family and some search members hated to accept what was more than likely a body recovery so several search teams were still hoping he would be found injured on the bank.

After working on a plan with Jim and other rangers we called in every swift water trained white water team we could find and began searching the entire gorge even with teams several miles down the creek towards Highway 30. As we had search teams busy, we began to expand our resources by requesting THP aviation and Beth Elliott who just happen to be flying with the Department of Forestry looking for fires from a fixed-wing Cessna. We requested at the time the only strong dive team we knew that also had an underwater camera capability (Knox County dive rescue team). I reached out to several folks and found a cadaver team out of North Georgia who was training in Chattanooga so we requested for their assistance. As with any search I also had a cache of TSP rangers assisting from bank search to Alan Wasik and Mark Morgan beginning to dive below Cane Creek Falls. I also requested ranger Dave Engebretson to assist with his kayak and he also brought several friends with him who had vast experience in white water and had floated this stretch before below the falls.

Without requesting a great friend of TSP was Mark Gribble who did our medical training for so many years traveled to Fall Creek with his new camera and videoed a lot of the search and interviewed many of the search team leaders and we were able to use this video for many years in Tennessee for search management training. Jim and I decided there was a great possibility the body was swept downstream and over the waterfall, so we began to put resources into this area that was almost impossible to access except for the steep "cable trail" which lead to the bottom of Cane creek falls so we decided to use reverse psychology to one of the smartest rangers I have known which was Robin Bayless!

We challenged Robin to see if he could get all of the tons of equipment we needed down the cable trail without killing anyone so Robin decided to use his years of Mountain rope rescue training to lower boats, motors, and dive equipment over the treacherous ledge at the Cane creek overlook. Robin spent a great deal of the night at the shop building a ramp/slide that would pivot like a teeter-totter to allow us to lower equipment from the top by the use of a 3 to 1 lowering rope system. As Robin began to lower the equipment with many of the maintenance personnel, we put much of our resources into the plunge pool below the falls.

Mark Morgan and Alan Wasik worked with the Knox County dive team in attempts to dive as much as they could under the falls however the turbulent water from the falls kept them away from the ledge just below the falls. Ray Cuthcher set up one of the most elaborate rope systems with Knox County that would allow us to systematically search a grid pattern with an underwater camera from a rubber Zodiac boat. During this same time, we swept the Cascades above the fall with the dog team with no luck as well as using the Chattanooga STARS team to check rocks and undercuts in the cascades area.

As the weekend was about to close and we knew we would lose a lot of our rescue squads since many must return to their paid jobs so, we knew we would have to rely on TSP rangers, so we began a rigorous dragging operation in the plunge pool as well as sending rangers downstream supervised by ranger Dennis Bayless. I ran home really quick to grab a change of clothes (this is when I found out you better keep plenty of underwear in your truck) but I also decided to give my Labrador (May) a try since I had been working on some cadaver material. When I returned to Fall Creek, I put May into the boat below the waterfall and began letting her work the pool and after a few hours, she seemed to show an alert several times in a small area.

I told Jim I felt confident in her alert but because I had never found a body with her and I did not want to alarm anyone or adjust the search plan we had for the day so I began my dragging operation just out of my curiosity that May might have made a positive hit on the body. During my dragging, I hooked something very large and heavy that I struggled to get up and before I got it up to the surface it became unhooked, and I never could get it hooked again so even though it was probably a large log but I will always wonder if I may have had the body for a few seconds.

Our operation was going into the second week, and everyone was becoming tired but when you see the families looking for you for answers you keep pushing onward in this instance the family believed the missing man could be revised with CPR after this long period so Jim and I decided to put together a communication plan that would stand for many years in TSP search tactics. Since the family was very close to our search area and radio communications were everywhere Jim and I decided we would come up with a code word for if the body is found. I had a green body bag with me so we knew it would be needed but also at the same time we spotted a set of old air splints in the Nature center so it was set; if the body was spotted search teams would call for a "Green Air Splint"!

Even though we felt we had put together a good search plan and had used a ton of resources we just could not find the body so we had to make the tough decision to scale back the operation and begin to try to re-open the park to somewhat normal format while still using rangers downstream. I believe Stuart or Robin had come up with the great idea to stretch a fence across the base of the plunge pool where the water would spill into the drainage for many miles. As our luck would have it on the day we took down the caution tape and opened up are seasonal ranger George Shinn led a group of young school kids to the overlook when the body surfaced. We loaded the body in the ambulance and took it to any area where the family and church members wanted a chance to "resurrect the dead" so we gave them time for this process and as of today, this was the largest and longest search in Tennessee state parks history.

SOUTH CUMBERLAND CARRY OUT

I was contacted one night by Park Manager John Christof concerning an abandoned vehicle found at the Fiery Gizzard parking lot for overnight hikers. The park manager stated the driver did not have an overnight permit and that he had contacted the girlfriend of the subject. She was very adamant that the man was distraught over several issues in his life, and she believed he had gone to the park to harm himself. When we pushed the woman for more information, we were able to get her to tell us he did not own any guns and would never try to shoot or cut himself!

We gave Addie a try and she seemed to work a small trail from the vehicle and continued all night until daylight when now and then showing some interest in an older scent trail. We had searched the entire Fiery Gizzard trail and were completely exhausted when we went to check on the Werner Point area when Addie lit up with her first ray of excitement toward the point. I noticed some colorful items at the base of the tree, but at first sight, it just seemed to be some clothing and gear. As we approached Addie investigated the clothing with enthusiasm and I pulled her back from the ledge and tied her to a tree while I inspected the site for any clues from the found items. Upon closer inspection, there was a pillow tied to the base of a tree, several cans of beer, and over a dozen empty packets that seemed to have contained some type of pills at one time. I began to carefully inspect the area but was also nervous because we were right on the side of a cliff at Werner Point.

I looked at the surroundings below the ledge where I spotted the man's lifeless body at the bottom. We later found a note to his family and deduced he leaned up as long as he could against the pillow while consuming beer and taking sleeping pills until he eventually fell off the cliff to his death from blunt trauma.

We contacted the local high-angle team (Coalmont) to assist us in roping down the side of the 100-foot cliff to package the patient into a Stokes basket and lift him back to the top of the cliff. At this point, the rope team only consisted of four folks and all of us were extremely worn out from the recovery and we had no idea how we would get the basket back to the parking lot with such a limited crew.

The rope team had to load all of their equipment and supplies back into storage and carry it out so they had their hands full and we only had four of us to make the several-mile trek! Next, you will read the most impressive action Addie ever performed on a search.

Park maintenance supervisor Carlton Parmeley knew the park as well as anyone and he knew a shortcut from Raven's Point that was only a mile or so from a farm that they used from time to time for rescues. I came up with the greatest idea ever in my entire career of searches!

We gave our packs to Carlton to carry out and asked him to drop his ball cap on the ground as he left the area and then we attached the all-terrain wheel to the basket that contained the body. Once we had the body ready for the carry out, I tied Addie to the basket and gave her the command to find Carlton and she tore out after him since she had a few hours of resting while we were retrieving the body. This was the most amazing sight to see that dog pulling the basket like a sled dog in Alaska and all we had to do was balance the basket all the way to the farm while following Carlton the entire way back. Another sad ending to a case but one of the stories I will cherish for my entire career!

- This case was taken from my first book "*Lost and Hound*".

SOUTH CUMBERLAND HYPOTHERMIA

In 2015 we were preparing to work another cold governor's inauguration when I received a call from park manager George Shinn concerning an overdue hiker at the Fiery Gizzard parking lot. The park was shorthanded due to several rangers out of state at training so, I mustered up what I could so many rangers from east and west had already responded to Henry Horton for the inauguration and did not have all of their gear with them but rangers all across the state did what they do, they responded.

Rangers at the park spent a long night on the trail clearing it and possible campsites while others did an outstanding job not only with the search but the investigation however, there were so many rabbit holes to run down. Rangers worked with the local police to gain access to the vehicle and began an inventory that produced his driver's license but the concerning item in the car was his backpack with essentials needed for a hike along with a map of the trail system.

Unfortunately, there was no answer, there was no answer on his cell phone, and it took a while to run down a house phone but no answer there either. The investigation by the city police showed he had used a credit card at a nearby market the day before so we know he was in the area but there was always a chance he parked the car and got in a vehicle with someone else and was in the ROW, (rest of the world). To give the rangers further confusion the car was rented so that led to a dead end. We contacted the Clarksville police department to do a welfare check at his apartment but no luck there and all of the neighbors said he pretty much kept to himself so, once again no luck.

What stuck out to me still to this day was a 10-pound box of yeast in his vehicle and that stuck with me as very odd I began to work with law enforcement partners up to the FBI on what he may be doing with the yeast! Could it be he was out in the woods making moonshine as they did there in the 1930s or was there a new type of drug on the market that he was trying to work out a new recipe for? I had made as many phone calls as I knew who to talk to when the park manager called me and said they got a hold of his employer and it turns out he was a "traveling yeast salesman", go figure!

At this time we were into the next day's search and I jumped in the helicopter with THP Lt. Brad Lund to look at every overlook and cliff edge in case he fell while rangers worked on clearing the top of the mountain inside the loop trail. At about this same time, his parents had reported him missing to Nashville Metro police, so we began a dialogue with them. His family said he was a frequent hiker but never overnight and our biggest concern at this point was he left his pack and extra clothing in the car and the weather was around 14 degrees. After a very long day of searching from the air and on the ground, we turned up nothing.

The next day we had to scale back a little since we were committed to security at the inauguration but there were still several rangers assisting one of the best backcountry rangers Jason Reynolds took it upon himself to look in an area that was off the park on private land and he brought the search to an end when he found his body. Our missing person had wonder off the trail and fell in the creek and with the conditions as they were he succumbed to the elements. All the rangers working that event, especially Jason are a perfect example of WHY GOD MADE RANGERS!

TRI CORNER KNOB HYPOTHERMIC HOIST

In early of the month of January of 2013 I was with my wife at Home Depot picking up items for our new home we were building when my phone rang from my friend and district lead ranger in the Great Smokie Mountains National Park Jared Saint-Clair and I knew he was not calling to say "hi"! He informed me they had been searching for an overdue hiker on the Appalachian Trail and rangers had just found his body in the Tri Corners shelter, which was believed to have been a death from hypothermia. The man had made it to the shelter but as in many cases of hypothermia, he had discarded much of his clothing and equipment along the trail.

The NPS ranges were asking if we could assist the rangers to carry the man's body from the shelter to the closest road which was a 15-mile trip! I knew this idea would take dozens of people and many hours if not days to cover that much ground in the mountains, however, the request got worse when Jared told me there were approximately 10 inches of snow on the ground! After getting this information I knew now why he called as it was going to take more people and time than I had originally thought about the extraction. I told Jared to give me a few minutes to work on a solution!

Knowing it was a long shot, I had been involved with a joint rescue program with the Tennessee Highway Patrol aviation unit where they had a new hoist on their Bell Huey. I explained the situation to Lt. Brad Lund knowing the risk involved in any rescue to save a life, but this was not to save a life but to hoist a fatality victim that posed a risk to our rangers in trying to get him out in the traditional method under these weather conditions. The decision was that the mission be used as a training flight since they had so many trainings per month.

We agreed to meet at the hanger at 6:00 a.m. the next morning, so I contacted the NPS rangers and laid out our plane. Several NPS backcountry rangers were staying at the shelter with their bodies so we would waste no time since there was good weather forecast the next day. Our crew of Brad, Captain Lee Chafin, Steve Manning, Jeff "Buck" Buchanan, and I loaded the Hughey on a very cold morning.

We flew to Gatlinburg airport to refuel and then headed to the Appalachian Trail to begin the recovery. As we hovered over our target (Tri Corners Knob shelter), Buck lowered Captain Chaffin down to the awaiting rangers. To save fuel and lower the noise for the recovery team Lt. Lund left the area which was a tight area. As we left the area we began to fly in the clouds at such a very high altitude when Brad banked the aircraft back to the mountain where there was a small clearing on top of the mountain on the Appalachian Trail and I made the mistake (and would make again on other flights) when I said "there is no way you can land in that spot! No quicker than it was out of my mouth we were landing in the snow on the A.T.!

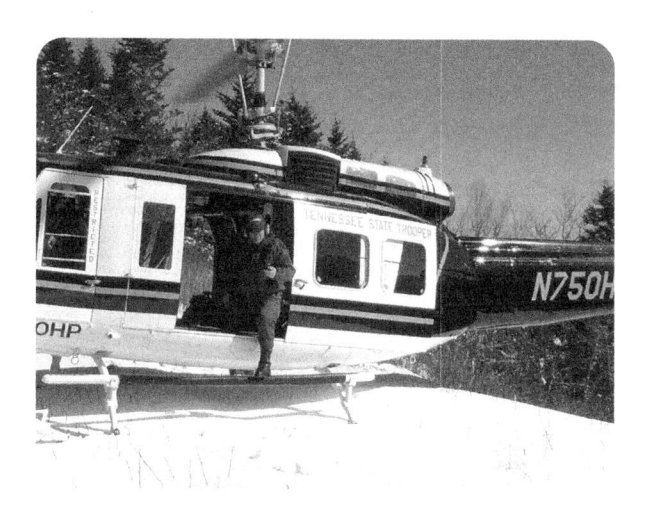

What I didn't know was the NPS rangers had cleared this area off the trail for this exact need! It would take a bit of time for them to package the subject, so we landed and waited for the call for the hoist. After we landed, it was too tempting for my partners in crime Steve Manning and Jefferey "Buck" Buchanan to exit the vehicle and have a quick snowball fight on the top of the smokies!

Soon the call came from Lt. Chaffin to return to the shelter and hoist the body up into the airaircraft, Brad lifted up and we circled over the shelter in the final stage to bring the hiker's body back to the family. After several minutes of a bumpy ride, we were able to safely return the hiker and Lt. Chaffin to the helicopter and we left for Gatlinburg airport where we would reunite the family with their loved one.

SNAGGING A TROOPER

In 2011 I responded to a drowning at Rock Island state park in which a man had fallen overboard while fishing. Park manager Damon Graham had begun search operations with several local agencies. Our biggest need was a side scan sonar and camera to find the body but in hindsight, the body was way above the point where the witness last reported seeing him go under but as in any crisis the human mind can be wrong s,,,,,o the information kept us downstream.

I brought in Tennessee Highway Patrol Special Operations troopers Steve Manning, Jeff "Buck" Buchanan, and my first meeting with Todd Greggory. I brought them in to assist with the need to dive and retrieve the body, but they also brought a small cheaper underwater camera than what we had on the scene I decided to use the camera upriver from the point last scene. I put the camera in a local rescue squad boat in the hands of ranger Scott Crick mainly due to the fact the local dive boat had damaged its sonar in the jagged rocks of the river.

As the ranger began searching above the PLS he yelled out "I saw the body" but we lost it again for a few minutes, so I instructed Scott to keep looking and requested THP troopers to begin putting on their dive suits. Troopers Jeff Buchanan, Todd Greggory, and Steve Manning entered the water and began a check off of their equipment when the body was once again spotted. Buck dove down several times before he finally found the body wedged between two rocks, so I put together a plan to retrieve the body.

Since the family and news service was on the far bank of the river, I decided the troopers would dive down and bring the body to the surface and the rescue boat would serve as a shield as they brought the body to me on the opposite bank and I would put the man into a body bag hopefully to protect the family from any grief. As Buck dove down trooper Manning was holding on to the front of the boat preparing to dive down and assist when all of a sudden, our entire scene was blown out of the water! One of the boat operators was moving from the rear of the boat to the from and tripped over a pike pole that had a 3-inch large treble hook attached to the end. When the man tripped, he accidentally forced the pike pole out the front of the boat and the hook pierced the nose of Trooper Manning!

When I use the word "pierced" I do not do Trooper Manning justice as I am sure he would say he was stabbed or snatched! Trooper Manning began a violent scream as soon as he was hooked and not only did the hook puncture his nose but it pierced all of the way through his nose the pole had upward pressure so it looked like it was pulling him out of the water like you would set the hook on a big fish! Right in the middle of Steve's plea for relief from the hook trooper, Buchanan surfaced with the body but due to the weight of the man Buck could barely keep himself and the drowned man at the surface so he began yelling for help from anyone who could grab the body from the boat!

My plan to bring the body quietly and methodically to the service to me certainly went out the window and I felt more helpless than I have ever been in my life with both troopers who were there to help me all of the sudden crying out desperately for my help as I sat helplessly on the bank! The view I was witnessing was nothing anyone can teach you in a textbook, but you react with what you have and hope for a safe outcome! Boat workers were able to grab the body and Buck attempted to help Steve and gain him some relief from the hook that still had him hog-tied like a sucker fish. Workers were able to cut the line attached to the hook in Steve's nose and Buck began bringing him to me, however, more drama was added to the scenario when Buck began inflating Steve's flotation device which caused too much pressure on his upper torso which also caused his new noise piercing to squirt blood in the air!

As soon as Buck got Steve to me, I grabbed him in my arms and he began demanding me to "yank the hook out of him" but I knew that would only cause serious damage and pain to my friend so I called for another rescue boat to transport him to the other side of the bank to the awaiting paramedics. As I drug Steve up on a rock in the water the rescue boat brought me the body and I attempted to put him in the body bag. Once we got Steve transported to the medical team, we floated the body down to the boat ramp at the beach for the coroner.

When I was sure all of the drama was over I turned to Trooper Greggory had been in the cold water for some time and began to realize he was in the beginning stages of hypothermia mainly due to the fact he was stiffening uncontrollably almost bouncing him off the rock back into the water. The Park Manager from Fall Creek was on the scene documenting the scene with his camera and I called him on his phone and asked him to take plenty of photos of Steve and his new attached appendage! Paramedics could not figure out what to do with the large hook when a local rescue squad leader went to his truck and grabbed a pair of large wire cutters and snipped the barb and removed the hook. As soon as we saw Steve smile over the ordeal, we were relieved but also began our barrage of jokes at his expense as law enforcement officers usually do with each other!

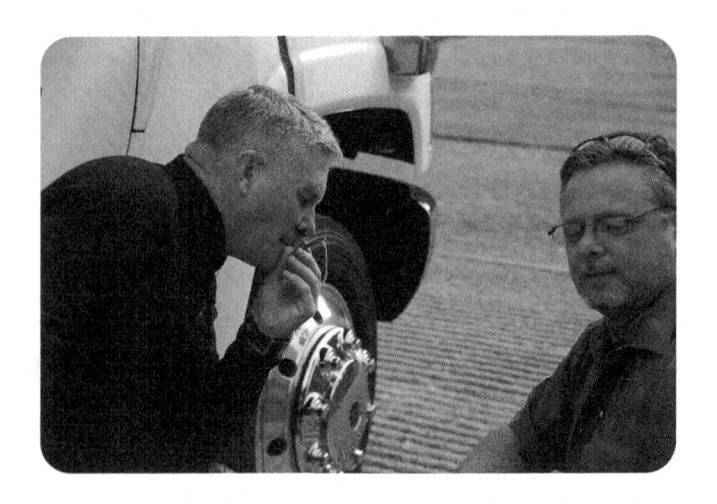

With the scene secure and demobilization complete, I called back to Lieutenant Ed Cherry over the Special Ops division and I told him "Lt. I have good news, your boys found the body for me"! I then asked Ed "Does the highway patrol allow nose piercing", and he said, "NO we do not"! I replied "sir looks like we are going to have to make an exception in this case", that is the bad news" My dear friend Steve Manning has reviewed and joked about this case for many years but words will never begin to express my sincere appreciation to him and the other members of their team!

SHELLY MOOK AND HOLY BOBO SEARCHES

2011 was a tough year for abductions in Tennessee, two of which I oversaw with TSP rangers assisting the Tennessee Bureau of Investigation on the missing women. Shelly was reported missing on February 25, 2011, from Bedford County after dropping off her child but was never seen again. It was and is highly suspected her estranged husband had brought harm to her back then but especially today as he has been jailed in Florida for his attempted harm to his girlfriend.

I approached TBI to assist them with our rangers to exercise the Incident Command system during our in-service training. I was able to organize approximately 100 rangers to search an area of interest for TBI in Bedford County in hopes of finding any evidence of her disappearance. The area was in a thickly wooded area just off the interstate but also had a large area of wetland swamp that would need to be searched.

Rangers were tasked with organizing, planning, and implementing all aspects of the search which entailed ground teams with boots on the ground as well as several rangers in kayaks and canoes to search the water. Unfortunately, we did not find any evidence that would assist with the investigation but every ranger got a lot of experience from that search and we left no stone unturned in the area for TBI and certainly for the family.

Holly Bobo was reported walking into the woods with a man in camouflage from her home in Darden Tennessee on April 13, 2011. I was contacted by local agencies if I could respond with my k-9 however I was at Fall Creek Falls on the firing range that day with my rangers, but I felt comforted knowing my friends with THP Special Ops and Craig Smith was on the scene with his bloodhound. Several very high-profile days went by with several agencies searching for Shelly both on the ground and in the air in and around the home.

5 or 6 days into the search TBI and TEMA asked if I could organize a search with rangers at Natchez Trace state park which was very close to the area of the home and seemed a high area of interest where someone may have tried to hide a body. I organized about 30 TSP rangers along with members of Tn. Division of Forestry and members of their law enforcement division as well as law enforcement officers from TWRA scouring the countryside of the 48,000-acre woodland. I had organized search teams to concentrate on the hundreds of miles of fire roads in the forest.

After two days of searching, we were requested by the same agencies to see if we could help organize the search for volunteers in wanted to assist in the process. Usually, this is the last thing we would do on a search since the volunteers are not trained or equipped for this type of search tactic and can contaminate or destroy evidence. Unfortunately, I was floored when the volunteers were sent to us in bus load after bus load with men, women, and children with many dressed in shorts and flip-flops.

The biggest issue that got the park manager's attention was the dozens of ATVs and horses that wanted to search the areas the park manager was losing his mind stating we don't allow this in the park which is a true statement, but I urged him we had to make an exception in this case due to media and public outcry.

We had to devote our ranger resources to the volunteers to ensure their safety but also keep any one of them from getting lost so we decided to use them on the roadways to look for evidence and the horses and ATVs on all of the trails. Many dead in hours of chasing poor leads and evidence from untrained individuals resulted in nothing but again we were able to let the family know we did all we could to bring Shelly home.

★On September 22, 2017, a jury found Zach guilty on all charges, including first-degree murder.[14] He was sentenced to life in prison plus 50 years on September 23. He maintains his innocence.[15] In January 2018, Zach›s brother, Dylan, accepted an Alford plea and he was sentenced to 35 years in prison.[16] Autry chose to make a deal with prosecutors wherein he would testify against Zach Adams in exchange for a significantly reduced sentence. On September 16, 2020, after accepting a plea deal that reduced his sentence to eight years of time served, Jason Autry was released from prison.[1]

SEARCHING FOR FRAN

One of the greatest women to have worked for the Tennessee Department of Environment and Conservation was Fran Walas. Fran was our staff attorney and not big as a minute, but she was a fireball when it came to legal issues and arguing the law! Fran was not only a champion for our parks and rangers, but she was an ambassador for all things environmental in Tennessee!

Fran was also very active with many park events and programs, but she was a very active and renowned hiker in Tennessee as well as other states. Fran knew many of our trails better than we did and she even wrote many articles for our departmental magazine *"The Tennessee Conservationist"* where she would rate the trail for difficulty and discuss its features to promote hiking to all!

Like many people who knew Fran, I very much admired her and had a special bond with her due to our jobs and safety issues in parks, however, I had one issue with Fran's hiking adventures since she almost always hiked alone and since I was over search and rescue for our park system and an avid search and rescue instructor I always urged anyone hiking to never go alone in case of an emergency.

Late one evening I was camping with my horse at Frozen Head state park for their Heritage festival the next day and

I decided to get some exercise for my horse and venture up the mountain on my steed. It was getting late, but I had all of my gear and radio packed so I told the ranger I would check a few overnight campsites to make sure the campers were all safe and at their registered site. After a few hours on the mountain, I was coming down to my camp when I noticed a single headlamp in the darkness and I thought a hiker may be lost since it was almost midnight, and who would ever have imagined behind the headlamp was Fran!

After a few cordial words, I told Fran I did not like her hiking alone and at night, and with Fran's beautiful smile she said, "I can do this hike blindfolded" and she was right on her ability and experience, but I was also right with the argument of an emergency. Also, in our relationship we both had a tremendous issue with a case we working on that was laying heavy on our minds and heart, so we spent several hours in discussion.

A few years later I received a call from another great employee of Parks, Jack Gilpin. Jack was also a dear friend to Fran and seemed to keep up with her adventures, so when he called me one down in a bit of a panic as to Fran's whereabouts, I took his call very seriously. It seemed Fran was hiking "somewhere" in the Great Smokey Mountains national park (by herself of course) and she had not returned to work or home! Her family had not heard from her and this was early in the days of cell phones and Fran did not have a phone for her person. Another pressing issue was that Fran had recently learned she had a heart valve issue, and this could have possibly been a contributing factor to her missing or overdue.

Jack gave me a few details but still, it was a shot in the dark as to where Fran could be in the 500,000-acre park! My big issue to begin with was no one knew her itinerary or which trailhead she may have begun and there are only 800 miles of trail in the smokies including 71 miles of the Appalachian trail running through the park! The only information I had going for me was Fran's vehicle description. Fortunately, due to so many searches that I had been on in the smokies I had made a great relationship with the rangers in the park. I immediately made a call to Chief Ranger, Dave Panabaker, and informed him of what we had, and for some reason, I felt she may be on the Appalachian Trail or one of its spurs.

Being such a fan of Fran and co-worker, I took her case very seriously, especially after learning about the medical issue which concerned us all! After alerting the national park I began to muster up several rangers in east Tennessee to respond to the park to assist as well as launching an airplane from the Tennessee Highway Patrol! As I began talking to family and friends of Fran, trying to somehow find a small clue as to her trail of choice the Chief Ranger called me and said they located her car at the New Found Gap parking area where the A.T. crosses the road.

Rangers from the park sprinted out onto the trail and within an hour they found Fran! She had gone down from a heart issue and couldn't make it out of the trail to her car, so when Rangers found her, they checked her out medically by their park medics then transported her out. This search wrapped up in a few hours and I can never thank the NPS staff for their professionalism in bringing our Fran back home!

*Tragically Fran died from injuries sustained in a freak accident fall in 2010 while staying overnight with a friend. The Tennessee Trails has a program in her memory where you can earn a "Fran Wallas" patch by hiking her 36 signature hikes! We all miss our friend!

A SEARCH AT ANDREWS KNOB

In mid-September, acting Chief Ranger Jared St, Clair requested a search crew to assist in a search for a 53-year-old Ohio woman who was missing in the Clingmans Dome area. Susan had gone hiking with her 20-year-old daughter on the Forney Ridge Trail headed to Andrews Knob. Susan's daughter wanted to make the trip to the top of Clingmans Dome but Susan wasn't up for the trek so they decided to meet back at the car in the parking lot.

National Park rangers were on their second day of searching and due to the vast area and cold weather conditions they began to reach out to many of the search and rescue partners they use on large-scale searches. They used approximately 175 trained SAR professionals from 5 states and 50 organizations but also used K-9 teams, drones, and helicopter support from the Tennessee Highway Patrol and Tennessee National Guard.

What was baffling by the search planners was the fact that the Forney Ridge trail is one of the most traveled in the smokies which also means the trail is beaten down and very hard to get off the trail. Several teams were already in the field when TSP rangers arrived, and the teams had hiked more than 500 miles of trail when the search was over covering about a ten-mile square search grid but no trace of Susan could be found.

I was sickened that I couldn't respond since I was just a week out from having surgery on a bone spur that had me pretty much crippled, however when Jared asked if I could work on getting THP's helicopter on the search I was eager to assist! I knew the area pretty well from several other searches in the area, especially the Phillip Roman search. We flew up on day 3 but the weather was soaked in with fog so thick that visibility was almost impossible from the air. I had asked Brad to concentrate on the drainage where Phillip was a forum and several other side drainages of the Appalachian Trail.

Due to the weather conditions and lack of overnight equipment and clothing, we were all concerned with the issue of Susan suffering from hypothermia. Search teams looked for Susan for the next week and on October 2nd her body was found in the Huggins Creek drainage which is a very steep and rugged drainage. It is not completely understood how or why she was in the location, but it is probable that she became disoriented in the darkness and began suffering from hypothermia. Somehow it is believed she missed the trail to the parking lot and ended up on the Appalachian Trail then into the drainage about two miles from the parking lot.

The NC State Bureau of Investigation joined in the search along with Christian Aid Ministries Search and Rescue, Gatlinburg Fire Department, Haywood County Search and Rescue, Oak Ridge National Laboratory, Tennessee Highway Patrol Rapid Response Team, Tennessee Search and Rescue Team, Tennessee State Parks, U.S. Forest Service

Cherokee Hotshots, as well as other National Park Service personnel from the Blue Ridge Parkway, Chickamauga and Chattanooga National Military Park, and Shenandoah National Park.

Other organizations aiding in the search included Backcountry Unit Search and Rescue, Black Diamond Search and Rescue, Blount County Rescue Squad, Blount County Special Operations Response Team, Blue and Gray Search and Rescue Dogs, Buncombe County Rescue Squad, Catons Chapel-Richardson Cove Volunteer Fire Department, Cherokee Indian Police Department, Cherokee Tribal EMS, Gatlinburg Police Department, and the Henderson County Rescue Squad.

SAD WRECKS ON THE HIGHWAY

One morning as I was headed to town a vehicle pulled out in front of another car and there was a terrible crash at the "Park Market". I immediately called for an ambulance and ran to the first vehicle where a lady was okay but her husband was screaming that she didn't even have a driver's license so I made it to the second vehicle which was an early model pickup truck with an older man behind the wheel.

The crash was very violent and the man inside was not responding to my voice so I was trying frantically to make access to him but neither door would open. At this time my friend 'Skinner" pulled up in the ambulance and came over to the truck and because of his vast experience with the trauma he was able to tell the man was dead and tried to calm me down that there was no need to try to get to him and I felt so helpless but there was nothing we could do without the proper extraction equipment.

A few years later I responded to a wreck on the southern border where two cars hit head-on late at night. I go there about the same time the ambulance arrived and I began to assist the medic with C.P.R. on a patient who was not alive. After a long attempt to bring him back, we had no success in getting a cardiac rhythm and he was losing a large amount of blood. We rushed over to assist the other paramedic to extract the other driver who was still alive.

Sometimes the job has very tough endings.

ROCK ISLAND BODY FLOAT RECOVERY

A man had drowned around the Twin Falls recreation area and TSP special operations teams were activated in attempts to locate and retrieve his body. We had used several rescue squad sonar and dive teams in attempts to locate his body. I brought in Maury County Tennessee EMA dive team to assist in diving the blue hole, which is where we believed the body was trapped in the bend of the river.

After several days of crews searching in multiple areas and with various devices (cameras, divers, cadaver dogs, kayakers, and drag teams) we had to make a decision that would halt the recovery efforts and possibly alter the entire search operation because TVA had stopped all generation of power to keep the water level low and safe for us to search, however after several days of this process TVA had to release water due to the rising of the lake above the dam. We had to agree to this request and pulled all our rescue personnel out of the gorge, however, we did request TVA to turn on all available generators to allow as much water to potentially and hopefully dislodge the body and push it downstream.

TVA released water all night long but did agree to stop generation for the morning to allow us time to make another search of the river gorge below the blue hole. I had instructed one of our best rangers in a kayak (Dave Engebretson) to put in at the twin falls at first daylight and float to the beach ramp to find the body. Not long after he passed the blue hole, ranger Engebretson radioed to me he needed a "green air splint", which is code for us that he had discovered the body on the island.

The park gets its name from the island just below the twin falls which is layered with large rocks, however when the dam is generating, the water almost completely covers the island but the decision to release all the water paid off in our search efforts with ranger Engebretson discovering the body sitting on the edge of the island. The search was over but now came the process to recover the body for the family, however, I had instructed crews to be on-site at 8:00 a.m. and the body had been discovered at 6:30 a.m.

Our other issue was the location of the body and the limited ability to get any rescue equipment or personnel to the area. There are no access points to the area by larger boats due to the shallow areas above the island and alongside the island from below and with the high water overnight the entire island was covered in mud making it very dangerous and almost impossible for crews to traverse the island from downstream. Unfortunately, in this line of work, you use all manmade and natural resources to locate and recover the body and the morning heat had brought vultures into the body. With just the two of us, I decided that we had not prepared or trained for it, but it was the only safe and viable option I could come up with to keep the environment and birds from the body.

I instructed Dave to paddle his kayak back up to the blue hole (400 yards) and I would meet him at the water's edge.

I made my way down to the water which is an arduous hike with only my PFD and a "Rescue Sked Stretcher System". As David made his way to me along the shoreline, I strapped on the Sked with the shoulder straps and climbed on the back of David's kayak and we began the trip back to the island. Even though David is one of the best boaters I know, I am sure he also has not trained to drag the Chief ranger on the back of his boat! As we traveled downstream the sun was getting hirer in the sky and the temperature was warming which only brought in more vultures.

As we finally made it to the island our mission now was to examine the body and confirm to the medical examiner it was okay to package the patient. I put the man in a body bag and then secured him into the sked. Fortunately, when I bought the sked, it was because it had floatation devices to use in this type of situation. Once we completed the packaging, I began to float the body downstream around the island to park manager Damon Graham and other rangers while David stayed with us for safety.

I must admit I had been to water rescue classes and was taught by the best to float downstream in swift water but never trying to guide a cadaver downstream tethered to me! As we carefully navigated the swift water around the island, I was happy to see Damon and others, from there we loaded him onto a rescue boat and David floated me to the boat ramp. Our mission was finally over after 4 long days.

RADNOR LAKE EMERGENCIES

One of the rangers I recruited early in my career that I am very proud of is Steve Ward. Steve took my role as a ranger when I left to be an assistant chief and after working for several parks he landed the job as park manager at Radnor Lake state natural area. We have worked very closely on several emergencies over the years statewide but also a few at Radnor Lake.

Late one afternoon I got a call from Steve that he had a suicide victim behind the visitors center and requested me to respond. I got to assist him as quickly as I could and we worked the sad case with Metro police for several hours before removing the body who had died from a single gunshot wound.

A few years later Steve called me with a similar issue of potential suicide, but we were not positive since there was a body in the lake. A family member had found a suicide note at their house from their dad who was suffering from cancer and the outcome did not look good. I responded to assist Steve and after searching the lake shore we found his body close to the spillway with workout weights tied around his neck. Another very sad day.

I had another call from Steve about a reported possible drowning in the lake. Once again I responded and found

Steve giving CPR to a man he had pulled from the lake. This was a very odd case since the is no swimming allowed. Steve had done a very heroic rescue/recovery from his training in water rescue and medical but unfortunately, our efforts to revive him were no good since he had been under too long.

POSITIVE IDENTIFICATION

Early in my career as a ranger, I began to know a young man who was sent to the park to do public service work by the court system which many times ends up being a "babysitting" chore, but this young man was a very hard worker, and I began to strike up a conversation with the young man.

I was able to learn after several days of him working he was a kid who just never got a "break" in life, his dad had been absent, and his mom didn't want him around, so he felt lost in life. Even though it was a sad situation the young man was an extremely hard worker and he kept quizzing me about being a ranger I told him I would do my best to get him a job with the park system, but he had to hold up his end of the bargain. He was very grateful for the opportunity, so I gave him my business card and told him to fill out an application, stay out of trouble, and stick to his education.

A few months had gone by, and I received a phone call in the early morning hours from the sheriff's department in which a deputy had worked a car crash between the park and Lewisburg at Highway 64 junction in which there was a fatality in the one car crash. The deputy went on to tell me that the subject was a young man, and he did not have any identification on his person, but the only thing of importance was he had my business card in his billfold!

The shock of the situation had me scratching my head about who this may be, and I was just not thinking straight that it was the young man who had done the public service work. I made the trip to the hospital morgue which seemed like an eternity to see if I could help with the identification and as soon as I viewed the body my knees buckled to know this kid who was finally about to get his life in a positive direction died by just missing a curve in the road.

Unfortunately, I could not recall the young man's name, so I had to go back to the park and find the paperwork and determine his name and phone number and then go assist the deputy with the notification of the next of kin. Truly a sad ending to a bizarre case and a life ended too early.

PLANE CRASH IN THE SMOKIES

On December 12, 2016, I got a text from the Tennessee chief ranger in charge of the Great Smokey Smokies National Park concerning an airplane that was overdue at the Gatlinburg airport. The pilot and his 7-year-old son along with his girlfriend had traveled from Florida to visit family in Tennessee for the Christmas holidays. It was believed from information the Federal Aviation Administration had passed on it was believed the small Cessna had gone down somewhere in the park but due to foul weather, the National Guard aviation was unable to fly to the area to look for the wreckage. I used our state texting system to request our search and rescue and ropes team to be on standby if we were needed.

Later that day the National Guard was able to fly and spotted the plane crumpled on a steep mountain cliff where it looked as if the plane was a few feet from making it over the mountain when it caught several trees. The Guard was able to determine there were no survivors in the plane it was too steep and the plane was too unstable on the cliff side. The NPS made an official request through TEMA for TSP rangers to be prepared for a very rugged accent to the aircraft. I summoned my group of rangers to meet me at the Little Pigeon River ranger station the next morning at 8:00 a.m. for a briefing.

Even though I had a good strong team the NPS chief decided he would make one team made up of NPS rangers and TSP rangers. The issue at hand was there was NO road access anywhere and the trek would take 6-9 hours with a 4,000 elevation climb. I strategically chose rangers with strong rescue and rope ability and one ranger (Mike Croley) who was a pilot and would be able to give technical advice on the scene. The team was loaded up and transported for their arduous climb that none of them will ever forget. Lead Ranger for the Smokies Jared St. Clair and I traveled to the Gatlinburg airport to meet with family members, the National Guard aviation unit, and a representative from the FAA.

As we were arriving at the airport so did the Blackhawk from McGee Tyson and I was relieved to see my friend Tracy Bantum who is an icon and hero on helicopter rescue for the National Guard! They were to stage at the airport until the rangers reported they had the airplane secure and bodies in the body bags to be hoisted out by the helicopter. As soon as we had our plan finalized we met with the family to brief them on our plan and then we met with the young man from the FAA who was fairly nice but at some point, he decided the bodies could not be moved until he had done an investigation. I immediately became upset and informed him it took our folks 8 hours to get there and it will take that same amount for them to return and unless he could hike to the scene ASAP were going to remove the bodies from the plane after all our folks had been through!

After several heated discussions, the question was brought up as to if the guard could lower him down to the crash scene but they said their protocols would not allow that so we were back to a Mexican standoff and I was ready to pull our guys off the mountain when the pilot made several calls to Washington to get approval and so they were finally able to take off and lower him down to investigate. As soon as he was finished rangers secured the aircraft to the mountainside and began the hardest job they will ever be requested. The girlfriend had been thrown from the plane and her legs amputated as well as her head; the child was fairly intact but obviously, he died from blunt trauma; the pilot had suffered a severe laceration to the head as well as a leg amputation. After the rangers had them in the bags Tracy was lowered down to haul the bodies one by one into the aircraft and bring them to the airport.

Back at the airport, we tried to prepare the family for the next actions, and unfortunately, as with any investigation, someone from the family had to identify all 3 bodies. As with our rangers earlier, it was one of the hardest things to open the bags and view the carnage for the family and then try to console them on their loss. TSP and National Park rangers began their descent down the mountain and the aircraft returned with an FAA official and all the rescue gear. As soon as we thought the night would slowly ease out of the way a call came in that a 10-year-old was missing on the boulevard trail on top of the mountain. Even though we were told it would take an extra request and aircraft to fly the mission the guard guys flew back that direction on their way to Knoxville and immediately found the child on the trail and kept a light on him until the dad was back reunited with him and they guided them back to their campsite, all in a day's work!

We returned to the little river ranger station and waited on our teams after a grueling 16-hour recovery they all came DRAGGING in with desperation on their face. I had their rooms at the motel and got them settled and then took them to get something to eat but it was late and I could not find anything open but waffle house so we ordered it smothered and covered and began to eat with the dozens of loud kids that were also inside the establishment. I will never forget a sight that came from Travis Bow as his head kept getting lower and lower until he fell asleep in his food!

Words will never be able to appreciate the HELL those rangers went through during that day and their service to mankind in their ability to bring those bodies off that mountain to the families.

PLANE CRASH AT FALL CREEK FALLS

October 23, 2003, I was awoken by a phone call from TEMA and this would be a first as they began to tell me that they received information from the FAA in Atlanta and Memphis that a plane went off the radar and the last coordinates were located to be Fall Creek Falls. What made the call more sobering was the issue that came from the other end of the line that the plane belonged to Bill Frist (at that time a U.S. Senator and speaker of the house) as well as a doctor and air to the Frist family health care. I immediately called the park manager Jim Hall and confirmed the information with him and told him I would be on the way and would meet him around 3:00 a.m.

As I drove my mind ran wild, if this was Bill Frist on this airplane I could only imagine the CNN news trucks and the F-15 fighters that would be sent thinking it may be a terrorist plot and I would have my hands full, however as daylight was breaking it was then determined that the plane belonged to the Frist family but it was an employee who was the lone occupant of the plane. As we worked with the local EMA and mapping of where the coordinates placed the plane we knew it may be in the park but not 100% positive. This was also my first time to meet a local THP Sgt. R.C. Christian who would later become a great friend after our paths crossed so many times and discovering how great a human can be in life!

As we were waiting on aviation search teams to fly at first light a call came in from some local loggers who had spotted the crash site on the back side of another friend Malcolm Jessup's farm which backed up to the park. As we were heading out the ambulance driver Jeff knew the property well and we decided he would take the lead so an ambulance, THP, and Jim drove hard and fast with lights and sirens raging, and as we drove down Highway 111 to the crash scene we were passed by a volunteer firefighter in his personal vehicle and small red light and I was soon to see another side of the THP Sargent! As we entered the land and drove as far back as we could we still could not find the crash scene. When we ran out of the area to drive, it was obvious the plane was just over the hillside and as I exited the vehicle I saw a crowd of volunteers running to the crash site R.C. hoped out of his vehicle and demanded everyone halt as THP was in charge of the scene and no one was allowed to the scene except myself to confirm there were no survivors.

This was my first plane crash to work and I was a little taken aback at the wreckage but also concerned that I could not find the pilot and knew there was no way he could have walked away from the crash but where was he? Upon further inspection, I was able to finally determine because the plane crashed nose into the ground and the pilot's body was completely obliterated by the engine and all I could find was a small part of the top of his head and brain matter. R.C. had made communication with the FAA and we were asked to guard the site until they arrived but it may take 24 hours for them to arrive. They did ask us to look for any clues that might help to determine the cause of the crash. It was obvious that the plane had crashed nose-first at full speed either from the pilot losing control or running out of fuel. As I scoured the area I will never forget the moment when I spotted an object in the woods and when I examined it further it was the fuel gauge on the plane and it showed empty!

Later that morning the pilot's father and brother showed up on the scene and wanted to see their loved one It fell on my shoulders to speak with them and urge them that the shell of their family member was gone and I did not want their last picture in their mind to be what was in that wreckage. We were able to turn over the scene to other THP troopers and I headed home from a scene I did not want to ever relive!

ANOTHER THP PILOT HERO
RYAN QUINN

I have been fortunate to have crossed paths with several pilots with the Tennessee highway patrol within my job as Chief ranger, mostly with search and rescue but also on many law enforcement manhunts and through the Governor's marijuana eradication program. One of the last pilots I worked with was Ryan Quinn in East Tennessee. Ryan became a trooper but he also served our state in another capacity as a pilot with the Tennessee National Guard, so I was glad he was re-stationed in East Tennessee since they had a vacancy in that region for several years.

Ryan is a great public servant and always has a big smile on his face but he also was quick to agree to work with us on looking at our east Tn. Parks and certain landing zones so we would be ready for future searches. One of the first calls we requested was from two missing hikers on the Cumberland Trail who had gone in at the North Chick trailhead and headed up towards Barker Camp but they did not show back up to their vehicle. Park manager Anthony Jones contacted me and stated they had two missing older hikers they were concerned with due to colder weather.

C.T. rangers had cleared the trail and nightfall fell with no sign of the two men rangers called off the search way into the night so I had Ryan set up to fly the next morning. As expected he was spot on with his timing to fly and made radio contact with rangers on the ground and then Ryan made several passes over the trail and massive natural area of 7000 acres. After an hour Ryan spotted the two men who had tried to hike out at night and got off the trail and spent a chilly night not prepared to camp. Ryan was able to contact rangers on the ground and talk them into the two men but also give me a call to tell me he made the find!

A year later I had another call from Anthony concerning some kayakers close to the same area who had gotten on water too high for their experience level and they didn't show up at their vehicles when expected. I contacted Ryan again and he was also quick to respond to our needs by flying over the area and the creek drainage but after a few hours, he could not find the boaters. He continued to fly the area taking a close look at the water in case there was an accident when all of a sudden he spotted the boats as he flew around taking a closer look at them but he could not find the boaters.

Ryan let us know where he spotted the kayaks and walked the rangers into the area when all of a sudden the missing boaters walked out from some brush near the boats. When asked why they didn't come out and make contact with the helicopter they said "We wondered what he was looking for"! Great job Sgt. Quinn!

In early May of 2021, I spent my last search with Ryan before retiring. On May 10 of 2021, I was contacted by park manager Josh Kuykendahl of the Cumberland Trail that they had a report from the wife of a man who had gone hiking at the pocket wilderness Laurel Snow trailhead in Rhea County. His vehicle was found in the parking lot by his wife when he was not returning home from a day hike with a neighbor's dog. Rangers took off in the night around 11:00 p.m. and searched all night both from the bottom and also access from the top but rangers had no contact with finding the hiker.

I requested more rangers from across the state to assist in the search and locals from Rhea County assisted the rangers during a day search. I requested assistance from Sgt. Quinn was on the SAR with aviation assets and as always he was on board. I was in east Tennessee on another investigation incident but agreed to meet him at the McGee Tyson airport and assist him in the aircraft as another pair of eyes. We flew to the search area and made radio contact with ground rangers and found them searching the creek banks since most of the trail had been checked multiple times.

The wind was pretty stout that day so Ryan had to spend a lot of time flying and watching powerlines in the area so I came to the main outlook. The area is a very deep mountain region where the trail starts at the bottom and leads to the summit so we spent much of our time trying to look at the cliff lines and below in case he had fallen. At one time I thought we had our man when I spotted movement down below but it was a fisherman who was on the creek upstream. We were called off for a bit for a road rage high-speed pursuit but the driver was driving so fast we could not get there in time to help the ground trooper so we returned to the search area. The day ended with no one having any luck in finding any clues, not even his dog.

Sgt. Quinn returned the next day while I was tied up with another situation and the search crews began to grow in size from neighboring counties as far as way as Chattanooga even reaching over 100 looking for our missing hiker. About 6 days into the search a household found the dog still tethered to his leash about 8 miles away from the search. The local sheriff and EMA moved the search to that area and began looking between the house and the pocket wilderness. After a few days of searching, it was determined that the dog somehow got away from the missing man and just ran till the family found him.

After 11 days a volunteer search party found his body between the overlook and the parking lot in a very deep and treacherous rock outcrop. It was believed he either got lost and wandered off the trail and fell in the darkness or possibly was trying to chase the dog when it may have gotten away from him and he fell during that act. Rangers and EMS partners worked to get his body out of the park.

PICKETT PARK PUP SEARCH

In 2019, park ranger Cameron Martin called our office to inform us he had a lady that was overdue from a hike. Her husband had called to say he had not heard back from her and her car was found in the parking lot of the hazard cave. She did tell her husband the trails she was going to hike which covered several trails in the park and she had two very large dogs with her so she should be easy to remember if other visitors had seen her. Cameron began to work the trails along with other rangers but as the day grew long she was nowhere to be found.

Assistant chief rangers J.R. Tinch and Travis Bow responded to assist the park with incident command especially since Travis had worked at the park for several years and knew it very well! The woman who was missing was the husband of a nearby county sheriff's deputy so he speared a lot of police search teams to assist. On the second day, I responded from middle Tennessee to the park hoping and expecting they would find her while I was on the road but things were not looking good as I grew closer to the park.

Cameron had gotten several reports from visitors that they had seen the woman with the two dogs at several areas in the park so it confirmed she had been all over the park but she could not be found in the park. We had several dozen crews in various areas of the park and it was a concern that she may have gotten lost either in the Pogue creek canyon area which is a very steep and rugged natural area adjacent to the park but there was also a chance she could have ventured onto the trails of the Big South Fork National Park and Recreation area trail system so the NPS rangers were assisting on the search.

As I was getting very close to the park I had a feeling she was going to be found possible just by walking down the road so I decided with the large number of crews in the woods I would cover several side roads in and around the national park. As I was entering the park I saw ranger Michael Hodge in the parking lot of the Hazard Cave parking lot with a lady and two dogs so I pulled in and ranger Hodge confirmed it was our missing hiker!

She stated she had finished hiking for the day but before leaving she would hike the Indian Rock House trail across the road from her vehicle, but the odd part of that hike is the trail is only .20 of a mile so it is just not an area a person would get lost on because it only takes a few minutes to hike to the rock house and back. Unfortunately, the lady made the bad choice to do some exploring off-trail when it ended so soon and she became disoriented and wandered into the state forest and portions of the national park.

When I checked her well-being, she was in good spirits and very embarrassed but her poor legs! She was wearing shorts and had a run-in with large briers and her legs were scared from top to bottom. She was even such a good sport she allowed me to take a photo of her legs to help remind folks to stay on the trail! Always a good outcome with the hiker finds us!

OUR WORSE RESCUE
CUMMINS FALLS FLOOD

I was at Cumberland Mountain state park assisting with interviews for a ranger position at Frozen Head state park that morning I made the biggest mistake an emergency manager can make when I was asked by the area manager, "How was the fourth"? The date was July 5, 2015, and I was proud when I replied "It was one of the quietest holiday weekends in a long time"! As we worked through the list of names through the interview process we came to meet David Brady who immediately impressed us with his resume and knowledge of the job when I received a text. I would never show disrespect to anyone during this process by spending time on my phone but because of the nature of my job, I must always babysit my phone 24/7 for the next emergency.

There are many people in the state of Tennessee I rely on in the toughest situations one of the most important is Lieutenant Brad Lund of the Tennessee Highway Patrol. Brad has answered my calls and text so many times in desperation for help during tense situations but today it was Brad calling me which is usually not an emergency so I text him and said I was tied up but "Do you have an emergency" and he replied "the worse we ever had, get to Cummins Falls". I hated to interrupt David during his interview but told the panel I had to take his call for there was something bad happening! I ran out the door by the lake to make a frantic call and when I reached the Lt. he said "We had a flash flood and there were a lot of people stranded and possibly drown at Cummins and I need you to get there immediately"! Brad has always been calm as a cucumber under the most serious of situations but I could tell in his voice this was bad. My reply to Brad was" Are you going to Nashville to get the Hughey to hoist them" and he stated, "If I don't do something now they will be swept away in 5 minutes they will drown"

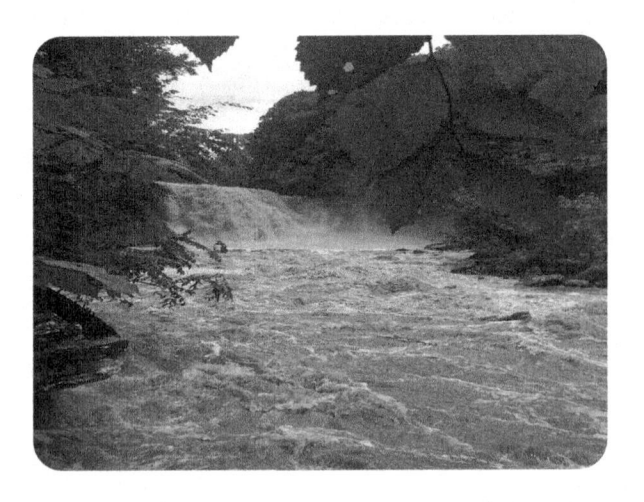

I lost contact with Brad and tried to call the manager and rangers but I knew they were at the bottom trying to rescue people! I walked back into the room and apologized for the interruption but also told the panel what a serious situation we had was and that I needed to leave as soon as we could wrap up the interview. We completed David's interview and

I knew I had to stay for the scoring process to ensure the legal transparency of the interview but my head was spinning of what was going on and what I needed to get for the park rangers! As soon as we were finished I told the park manager of Frozen Head Dave Engebretson I needed him as soon as possible at Cummins and I was so glad he had his kayak in the truck with him. Over my career, I have worked thousands of emergencies and for so many of them, David has always been there for me due to the fact he has always been the best hiker, backcountry search ranger, and an expert on white water in his kayak! I trusted Dave and his talents as much as anyone in the park system and I knew he would be invaluable on this water emergency!

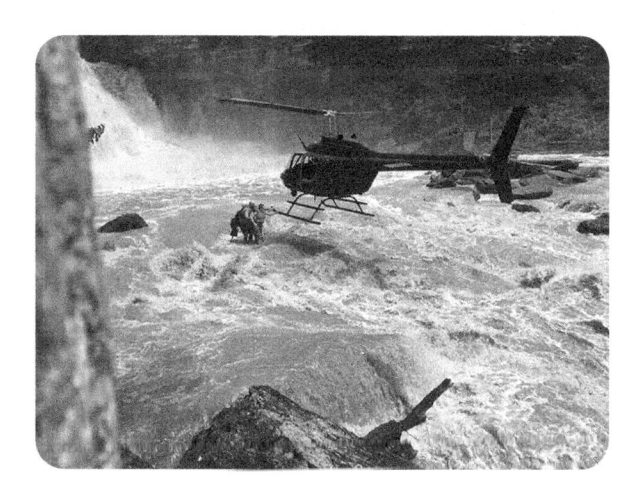

As I drove hurriedly down the interstate I was making as many calls as I could to get help and resources to the park but with little information, I had little to go on! I made contact with the emergency operations center at TEMA and they informed me there was a serious flash flood upstream from the park and flood waters had entered the park and swept dozens of parkgoers downstream! They also told me that THP was attempting to rescue people and they were trying to decide if they needed to launch rescue Blackhawks from Knoxville. I continued my route to the park and finally got a call from ranger Ashley Clark and found out she was off that day but I needed her at the park to stay on top to get me information on the situation! I then got in touch with rangers from Standing Stone and requested them to the park for support!

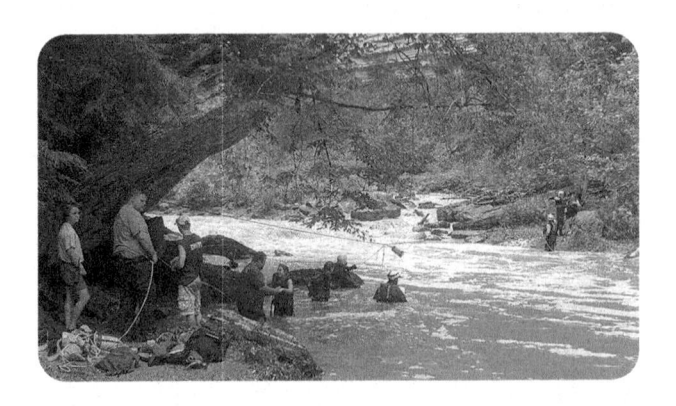

As I was coming through Cookeville Ashley reported back to me that rangers had set up a rope system across the water and were walking people across the stream that were stranded on the island. She also told me a helicopter was attempting to fly down into the gorge and rescue several folks who were clinging for their lives on a rock in the middle of the flood water below the falls! I finally made it to the park and Ashley briefed me on the situation that the pilot had somehow flown down and rescued an entire family one by one who was certainly about to drown after so many minutes clinging onto a rock huddled together and holding on for their lives waiting on a miracle!

Since the first day I heard of Cummins Falls I was concerned about the safety of the park so after a long few days of rope and helicopter rescue training with THP and TSP rangers I asked Lt. Lund if he could fly us over in the Hughey to see if we could perform a hoist operation down in the gorge if some type of emergency happened. As we flew over the tiny gorge I was a little apprehensive about easing down into the gorge but I have the greatest trust and admiration for Brad Lund and his abilities in a helicopter. Lt. Lund and his Captain over the hoist Lee Chaffin both agreed it would be tough but they could do a hoist if needed. Over the next few months, Brad and I would discuss what abilities and resources we could use in case of an emergency. Brad told me he thought he could land down in the gorge with a smaller aircraft if possible so we could load a patient out and I made my first mistake of challenging my friend by saying "I just don't know if you can get down in that gorge with your Bell ranger, there is nowhere to land"! I knew I had thrown down the gauntlet to challenge my friend but I did not think he could get the lift out of that hole, so late one summer evening as many days in Tennessee several thunderstorms moved through the state and it caused rangers at Cummins Falls to evacuate the park early and as timing would have it Brad just happened to be flying over the park late that evening and noticed the park had been closed up for the day so here was his chance.

Later that evening I received a text from Brad with no message but just a photo from my friend with a THP Bell helicopter sitting on the sandbar with the falls in the background. I just smiled thinking of what was going through his mind as he sent that message to me only to say "Don't ever say I can't do something! Of course that was not the case but it shows the outstanding professionalism and dedication Brad has to rescue operations in Tennessee. He and I both knew it was just a matter of time before we had a bad emergency in the park so he was just taking the next step to prepare. Later that year he gave me a call and we joked over the photo but he wanted to take the next step in preparing for a water emergency. He told me to meet him at AEDC where there were going to be doing some night operations training but he had a few hours that afternoon so he wanted to once again prepare for a water emergency. We took advantage of the afternoon with no interruptions so Brad would fly low on some train shipping containers and we would practice me getting out of the aircraft while he hovered with one skid on the box car while I would load a practice rescue dummy in the back. After we mastered that skill we practiced doing a short haul with the same rescue dummy in a SKED rescue basket. We continued this training until dark and went on our separate ways believing we had taken that next step for rescues but nothing would ever prepare us for the next rescue.

Miracles come in odd packages and many may not believe in them but this day was a miracle because it just happen by chance that the worse flash flood in history trapping so many people on rocks Brad was also in the area after working an armed robbery in a nearby county so he got a call from TEMA to see if he could get eyes on the situation and when he did make it to the park he could not believe his eyes and he had never seen that falls this big but also he spotted several folks up on high ground trapped but safe and then he noticed a true emergency when he spotted several people huddled on a rock arm in arm while the raging flood water were beating them every second in attempts to sweep them away.

OUR FIRST ACCIDENT INVESTIGATION

I was a very young new assistant chief ranger picked by my boss Ed Schoenberger when we were notified of one of the most tragic accidents ever at Fall Creek Falls. It was the spring of 1995 when a group of about 100 kids went on a field trip to Fall Creek Falls state park even though the kids were well supervised they were excited to explore the park so, after unloading the bus they raced to the falls. Many explored the view from the top when several were allowed to go to the bottom of the falls, which is a strenuous trek but no match for a young teenager.

Several of the kids took the trail that led above and across the creek that led to the falls but two of the young ladies from the trip made a bad decision and explored the top of the falls. Unfortunately, this is a common practice for many people seeking a thrill even though the park has many bright red signs stating "DO NOT ENTER, DANGEROUS FALLS AHEAD"! The girls crossed the sign which is a fence to encourage thrill seekers from entering at this access point.

The falls are controlled by the park from the lake so, depending on how much rain the region has experienced more water that will be coming over the falls so on this day the valve was open to full capacity to allow enough water to leave the lake so it does not get too high. As the girls got to the creek it is not sure why they still decided to cross the swollen fast-moving creek but just a bad decision in nature. It is presumed they wanted to get to the top of the falls for a better look at the gorge on the other side which gives a more open view of the falls.

One of the girls entered the swift water when she was immediately swept downstream, and she screamed for help from her friend, and when the second girl reached to help she was drug into the water as well. They were only a few dozen feet above the top, so time and swift water did not allow them the chance to get out of the water and they were swept over the 256-foot waterfall. Rangers were immediately contacted and several responded along with local responders. Sadly, one of the girls died from the fall but one of them somehow survived the horrific ordeal.

Not to take away anything from any of the responders but I am reminded of the heroic selfish actions of then-park interpretive specialist Stuart Carroll who raced to the bottom with scuba gear and spent time in the frigid water below the fall to eventually recover the body of the second young lady.

The one young woman who survived was rushed to Erlanger Hospital where she went through a long recovery from multiple injuries. Many people ask and demand we make the park safer there are always steps to add more signs but unfortunately, thrill seekers have and will always bushwack new ways to access dangerous areas. These bushwacking tactics allow a path for others to trek down into these areas. Park rangers at Fall Creek have spent countless hours pulling brushes to deter these homemade trails and added signage but we all have to educate all of our friends and family of the dangers of an unforgiven wild area.

In my career, I have been to the park hundreds of times, and on every trip, I make time to see the falls my mind always goes back to the day the girls went over the falls and it breaks my heart to think of the impact it had on so many lives.

Please practice safe hiking!

MY TOUGHEST DAY

Late one evening I got that call that I have received so many times before that comes with the job as Chief Ranger; that call that someone has died in a park! This night it was the park manager from South Cumberland state park John Christof, who proceeded to tell me had a death when a young man had jumped from a waterfall and broken his neck. I went through the motion as I had done so many times before to record the information of who, what, when and as I asked if they had gotten in touch with the family they replied no but they had been trying for several hours.

As I went down the check-off sheet of the name John said the name of the young man and his address was from my hometown and my heart sank! Every fatality I have been involved with takes a little from me but tonight it hit hard and personal. I was not close to the family but knew of them and also had the information they were a great close-knit "God-fearing" clan. I immediately told them to stop the phone calls and that I would do this in person, so I called my pastor whom we went to church as I knew also he was close to the family as well. On the phone, I told my pastor I needed his help on this one, and when I told him who the individual was he did not hesitate to say he would be there with me! He also told me he knew that the dad was not home as he was at a college awards banquet in Nashville since they had spoken earlier in the week.

I drove to my hometown one county over and picked up my friend and we made that short but slow-motion drive to the house. The next information still haunts me to date and I will never get it out of my head; as we exited the vehicle and began to walk up the winding sidewalk I spotted what would break my heart! Through the open front window, I could see the dad who was having a jokingly last-minute discussion with his son before they turned in for the night and I knew my next actions would change his life forever. I turned to my pastor and told him "I couldn't do this" and his wonderful encouragement gave me the courage to take the next steps.

As I approached the door and gave that knock I wanted to escape so bad so I did not have to deliver what would soon be coming out of my mouth. As the dad opened the door he looked at me in uniform and then my pastor and……he knew! He looked at me and said, "My son died jumping off that waterfall didn't he"? I could find the words and I didn't have to as he could see it on our faces. His emotions took over and this is the toughest time in anyone's life to have to deliver this information because there are just no words of comfort during this time. We sat on the couch and discussed the accident and what happens next to begin the grieving process and how to bring his son home for the last time.

I have had to make this notification several times in my career but this was certainly the hardest and most personal. This event still visits me in my mind and the view of that long trek up the walkway will always be my worst day!

MY FIRST RESCUE

We have a saying that rangers "wear many hats" and this day was a perfect example of how diverse our job can be! It was my first Thanksgiving Day to work at my new park which was known as a hospitality park which meant it had several amenities including a restaurant and my manager expected everyone to pitch in to make the visitor's visit a great one! My job today was slicing key lime pie when we received a call from the sheriff's department for us to respond to a spot on the river a mile or so from the park that was a local favorite hangout for folks and usually was met with alcohol in tow.

The information came to us as a male subject had fallen into the river from a rock bluff and there was another man and woman present. The park manager Eddie Schoenberger told me to jump in and we grabbed our rope equipment and basket and responded to the scene. The man had been underwater for a while but due to the cool water, there was still a chance we could revive him. Eddie and I rappelled down the cliff where the witness stated he entered the water but we could not spot the subject because the river is pretty deep in this spot but rescue squad members were able to hook the body and bring him to the service.

Eddie and I began CPR immediately as well as packaging the patient in a basket and began to get him to the top and continue CPR as we put him into the waiting ambulance.

Unfortunately, this was also my first encounter with CPR and body fluids of blood from the trauma of the fall. As we were headed back to the park we were given the bad information that this subject was a hick risk individual and we should decontaminate as soon as we could so we returned to the maintenance and stripped down to our birthday suits and began a straight bleach bath in hopes to remove any body fluids.

Unfortunately, this was also my first fatality as a park ranger, hate we couldn't do more!

MONTGOMERY BELL LAKE FIND

This story is a follow-up from my first book "Lost and Hound" in which ranger Eric Runkle at Montgomery Bell contacted me about a vehicle found abandoned at the Woodhaven Lake boat ramp. Ranger Runkle informed me it was registered to a lady from a neighboring county. The car had been there all day so I was asked to come in to see if I could run a trail with my bloodhound.

It took a few hours for me to get to the park with my K-9 partner and we made entry into the car to retrieve a scent article. We began the search and Scout trailed in a few circles and then began a track along the trail which ran aside the lake. After a few minutes, Scout alerted in an area close to the lake where we found a newspaper on the base of a stump and then the dog led me to the edge of the water making an indication the scent went into the water.

I let her cast in a circle to pick up the trail and once again she took me back to the edge of the water and gave me that look "Boss our person went in the water right here"! After further inspection, I found disturbance and evidence that someone had entered the water, so I was positive our individual from the vehicle was in the water. At about the same time we received information from the sheriff's department that the individual belonging to the car was wanted on charges from out of state and detectives were flying to talk.

I wasn't sure what action to take next so I called my hero from THP pilot Brad Lund to see if he could assist with a fly over the lake in search of our missing person in the lake but hopefully, they had made it back on land. I met Brad at the ball field next to the campground and we took off to get a visual of the lake and park from the air. We covered the rest of the trail that led around the lake with no visual contact so we began to search for the waterway. As we returned to the location the dog had led me to the water's edge Brad suddenly said, "There is your body"!

The victim had started to float, which was surprising since the water was still pretty cool letting me know the body had probably been in the lake longer than we thought. This find was a great example of using all of the "tools in the toolbox" that we teach in missing person cases; investigation, k-9, man tracking, and aviation support.

MIRACLE IN THE MOUNTAINS

The call came in on a very cold day in December for the request to assist rangers in the Great Smoky Mountains for a missing college student on the Rainbow Falls hiking trail area. I immediately began working to muster a rescue team but most of us feared it would be a body recovery due to the fact the temperatures had been hovering around 20* for the high and teens at night but those would be high compared to the elevation of the mountains in East Tennessee! My call out was complete and for so many times in my career, we headed to meet at the Norma Dan (a hotel that was locally owned in Pigeon Forge and worked closely to take care of search teams when the Smokies called)!

"I went to the overlook of Rainbow Falls and the 3 other friends who were with me went on to the top to the actual falls and I yelled to them I will meet you here at the junction when you come down the trail". That would be the last communication she would have with any human being and the beginning of the fight of her life! (Jennifer Dates interview May 7, 2020).

As Jennifer waited for the rest of her hiking team to return from the falls she began to be concerned that darkness would make the trek down to the parking lot a bit difficult. What Jennifer did not know her friends thought she yelled back to them that she would meet them at the parking lot so; as they made the descent down from Rainbow Falls they mistakenly passed and left Jennifer at the overlook. Jennifer decided to make the climb the rest of the way to the top to find her friends but discovered they were not there at this point Jennifer realized her party left without her and if she was going to make it back before dark she would have to hustle down the mountain! As Jennifer began the descent she had no idea that the 3-mile hike to the parking lot would take 2 days and bring her body to the point of death from freezing temperatures.

As Jennifer began her hike she pulled out her flashlight to find the trail and her worries mounted as it began to rain she thought in her mind could it get any worse when her flashlight began to fade from either the dampness from the rain or the batteries just weren't strong enough to throw a beam for her to find the trail. If you have ever hiked trails in the mountains you know there are many "switchbacks" that zig-zag the steep terrain and on this trip, after her flashlight went dead, and accidentally missed the switchback. This mistake lead her into the darkness and then a fall into the water from the falls that would begin her nightmare in the mountains!

If you are not aware of the requirement for hypothermia to the body there must be 3 elements; cool weather, moisture, and wind. I have been on several rescues that turned into body recoveries due to hypothermia and with no disrespect to Jennifer we all believed her fate was headed down this path. Certainly, Jennifer's body was beginning the process of hypothermia by adding moisture from falling into the creek, and if you have ever spent any time in the mountains you know the wind always blows and on this night the temperature would reach down to 5 degrees and the wind chill to -11*! Jennifer's 40-hour ordeal of hell was only beginning.

Jennifer spent the next day trying to make her way down the mountain but her body would not function the way she wanted it to from the fall and pending hypothermia leading to her possible death. At this point search teams from the national park were assembling a large-scale search for Jennifer and I was on my way from middle Tennessee with a load of TSP rangers, unfortunately, we would not make it to the mountains until dark and we were hoping the smokies rangers would have good news of finding her but no luck of finding Jennifer and we were heartbroken of knowing if she was still alive the night would take her from this earth!

So God Made Rangers

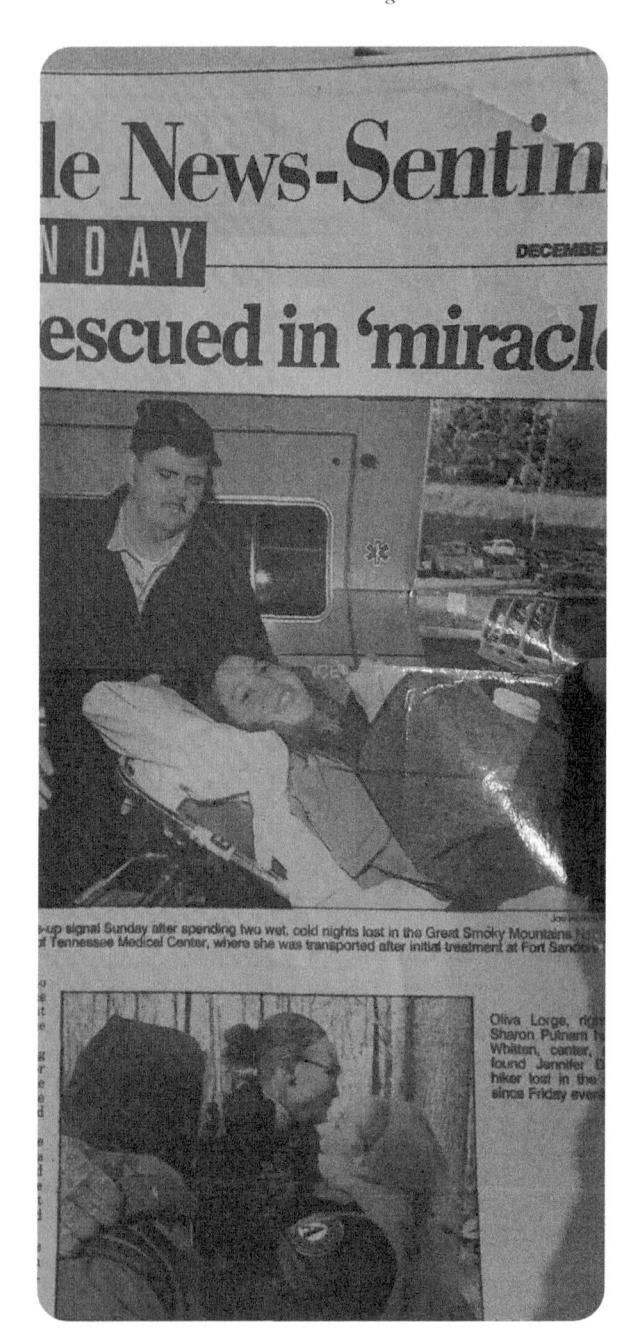

When I teach children my Hug a Tree program of how to survive in the woods I always ask them if "Have anyone of you ever had hypothermia"? I then begin to tell them how they have all had it if they have goosebumps which is the first sign of hypothermia. Jennifer became scared as night fell again and her body began to shake violently from shivering in an attempt to create warmth and friction from her muscles to keep her body temperature from falling. During the night Jennifer began to taste death and hallucinate from hypothermia and then began to throw up bile that she stated "tasted like death".

It is very hard for me to put in writing what Jennifer told me about the next night and what went through her mind. She began to have so many emotions go through her head and thoughts of how to die. As she lay on the cold ground and her body shaking she made the decision that NONE of us can ever imagine! She realized she was dying a slow death and so she would begin to remove the frozen clothes from her body and lay on the ground to speed up the process of death and put her out of her pain! As she lay there on the hard ground her mind began to wonder and she saw an image of her mom being told by rangers that she was found dead with her clothes off and she realized she had to fight for her life so her mom would not have to spend the rest of her life with that thought of her baby girl laying on the ground.

She sat up and put her wet cold clothes back on and she was shivering so bad she could barely get them on her body but the cheap "Wal-Mart" fleece and Vasque boots in their wet condition helped to keep her warm enough to make it to see the sun rise again! Jennifer huddled under a tree with her fleece pulled over her head and arms inside like a cocoon. As the sun rose and her body began to show a small bit of life Jennifer attempted to walk on her frozen feet in another attempt to find her way out!

At this point, I was several miles up Rainbow Falls hiking trail with a group of TSP rangers on my hands and knees under mountain laurel attempting to find any clues of Jennifer. I remember being cold and wet and making the statement there is no way this girl could have made it through this alive when a call came over the radio she had been found. As Jennifer attempted to walk she spotted someone who ended up being an Ameri-Corp worker for the National Park and a member of the search team looking for her. Jennifer was only a few hundred yards from the Rainbow Trailhead parking when she was found!

As we hustled down the mountain we still had no clue if she was alive or dead or any information on her condition! As I found my way to the parking lot and saw a lot of smiling faces I noticed something in the parking lot and made my over to the object when I realized it was Jennifer's shoes and socks. As I picked up her socks they were as hard as a board and I knew even though she survived she would lose most of her toes.

For many years this search would cross my mind and I always wondered how she survived I knew it had to be a great story so I began my research to find out who this girl was and did any of my old ranger friends in the smokies remember the search. After my go-to on all Smokey searches, Bob Wightman couldn't recall the search I was a little worried but after he contacted former chief ranger Steve

Kloester he brought it up to Helen McNutt and she remembered Jennifer's first name right off the bat! I wanted to interview Jennifer but also let her know how many kids I educated over the years of the seriousness of hypothermia and how great a fleece jacket can be in insulating the body even when it is wet and cold. Since that day I also made sure that every park ranger jacket even up to today is made of polar fleece!

When I finally got to interview Jennifer in May of 2020 I was so impressed with her courage and her will to stay alive but also could not believe her story up to today! When I asked how many toes she lost to frostbite she said "Well none but it is a long story". Both feet became swollen with infection and doctors had prepared her that she would probably lose her toes and possibly her feet in great Jennifer courage she was so glad to be alive she didn't care if they took off her feet! Her parents brought in a frostbite specialist who worked with various therapies and saved her feet! It was very interesting to hear her tell me that she can snow ski and do any outdoor activities as well as anyone, however, she said when she goes to the beach and lays out in the sun her feet get cold, and when she snow skis her feet get hot!

It is certainly a miracle that Jennifer is around to tell this story as a normal person would not have survived this ordeal! I was very proud to have played a very small part in this search but it is certainly why we rangers and rescue personnel do what we do! Thanks to God for sparing Jennifer to tell her story and inspire and educate so many young outdoor enthusiasts!

HARRISON BAY WIDOW MAKER

You never like getting that call at 2:00 a.m. but my career brought hundreds but this one was as tough as it gets. Long-time ranger and park manager Don Campbell who is an icon with state parks but this night was one of his toughest. There was a bad storm that came through the state with incredibly high winds and the top of a tree broke off about 75 feet in the air and fell on a tent.

As sad as it is to tell it was a husband and wife that were tent camping and the large limb fell on the man and he was found deceased in the tent by Don. I knew this was a tough scene for Don so I immediately jumped in the truck and raced to Hamilton County to help with the investigation and to be there for Don and the family.

Rangers do wear many hats such as medical but it is hard to prepare for situations such as this we also are safety officers and try our best to mitigate these types of accidents by inspecting trees and limbs for this exact emergency. After I got there I helped Don to take down the tent and equipment for the family and work with the sheriff's department on the investigation. Unfortunately, the limb was not a dead one waiting to fall but a perfectly live tree but due to the storm, it was torn off.

These types of accidents are referred to by some folks as an "act of God" but it is a very tough and depressing part of the job that sticks with you forever. This is a perfect example of why I have so much admiration for what rangers like Don have spent their career serving the public in need.

GREETER FALLS MISSING PERSON

In 2021 I was contacted by assistant park manager Bill Knapp from South Cumberland state park that they had a missing person possibly in the greeter falls area of the park. The family of a local man stated he spent a lot of time in the area and it was suspected he may be in the park area possibly searching for ginseng. As rangers were searching the area they found some items belonging to the man such as a small digging shovel that confirmed their suspicion of possible illegal activities but after a long day of searching the man was still not found in the park or at his home.

Bill had requested if I could assist with the THP aviation unit so like many times before I called my friend Lt. Brad Lund for help. Luckily he said he had some time the next day so I met him at the hangar to fly to the park and see if we can assist with the search. We got there mid-morning as soon as the fog burnt off and joined the search while rangers searched on the ground. Brad showed me the new FLIR system on the aircraft and how it could be used during the day to find the heat from an individual.

The drainage below the falls was a very steep and rugged area so searching on the ground was very slow and treacherous for those on the ground but it also made it difficult from the air. Even though the time of year played to our favor with no leaves on the trees but the sun was throwing too much glare for the FLIR to give us much help. We continued to give support from the air looking on top of the gorge but also deep down in the creek drainage.

After a few hours of searching, Bill said they had found a "rock house" where someone had drug some living equipment to make a small camping area on the side of a cliff and he asked if we could take a look at it. We flew to the area but because of the location in the trees, we could not get a close enough look at the shelter to determine if we could find anyone in the shelter. A few minutes later Bill said they could see a person's feet but the individual was not responding to their verbal commands nor was he moving. After a bit of time, law enforcement rangers made their way to the shelter and made contact with a man who was the missing subject we were looking for.

He had taken a fall and was injured and made his way to the shelter by coincidence and was trying to mend himself or just rest. Rangers then do what they do best and change hats from now a search rangers to now a rescue and recovery ranger. Once decided they would use local resources to carry him out Brad and I flew back to Nashville. Kudos to the South Cumberland Rangers for finding this subject and more than likely saving his life.

FORT LOUDOUN STATE OF EMERGENCY

I received a call from park manager Joe Distretti late one Friday night about an issue he was having in the park. They were hosting a very large boy scout jamboree with several thousand scouts and families in a backfield but a very large storm front moved in that evening and night dropping several inches of rain and to make things worse there was a cold front behind the rain. Joe was extremely concerned about the kids becoming hypothermic from the moisture and bitter cold.

Even though the above information is all true you needed to know Joe D! He was an old military man, but he also could blow some situations out of proportion! I responded and requested several rangers from across the state to assist to see what if anything we could do!

One of the biggest issues Joe informed was the area had no real road access to the open fields and the large amount of rain had saturated the ground and the cars were all getting stuck trying to get up a hill and out to the main road. In normal Joe fashion he was requesting rangers to ring equipment to make a gravel road to get them out so, Robert Wood came up from Nathan Bedford and did what he did best and that was running a loader.

There were two hilarious things I remember from the day as soon as I got there; first Joe was running around claiming he was "declaring a state of emergency" like his head was cut off and the second was my close friend Jeff Wells walking down the road soaking wet with a big smile on his face! I told Jeff we needed to calm Joe down and Jeff wished me luck on that so, I told Joe "Only the governor can declare a state of emergency" and we were not going to call him!

After we began to look at the situation the one true thing was that the cars could not get up the hill due to mud and the more cars drove the more mud ruts they made. Even though the correct weather was present for hypothermic emergencies it did not seem to bother the kids! Most of them were out running around or playing football in the mud while the dads were packing up as they were ready to leave.

Joe had ordered dozens of loads of gravel for Robert to make a new gravel road to the highway but rangers were going to still tow every car up the hill to the new gravel road. Jeff and I came up with a sketch that would be a little sketchy but believed it would work! We found a downhill route that would take the cars to the park road but it was a very steep hill on the way down. We told the drivers we had a route but they were on their own since the hill was so steep and it would only get slicker after each car traveled down the hill!

The first vehicle was released and our plan was working but as we expected about a dozen cars traveled the route and it became as slick as glass to the point cars were sliding so fast it was about to get too dangerous. Just as Jeff and I were about to shut the cars down due to dangerous situations Robert had completed his gravel road. Many of the miserable scouts and families left but those who were prepared decided to stay and make the best of it, after all, they were scouts!!

Still to this day every time I enter the park I look at that hill and just smile on the day we had a state of emergency!

FALL CREEK TRAGEDY

In the spring of 2017, I received a call from the park manager at Fall Creek that they had a fatality in which a ten-year-old had fallen off from one of the overlooks at the Falls. A father had taken his daughters to the park to see waterfalls but unfortunately, he picked a spot off the trail close to the cliff edge to have a picnic lunch when they were finished the little girl was excited to continue down the trail to the falls but before the dad could do or say anything this precious soul of a child went the wrong way and off the edge to a 200 plus footfall.

Of course, the rangers and rescue personnel once again do what they do to respond so by the time they had to call me the incident was well on the way. At this time it was about 9:00 at night and I immediately told my wife and supervisor I was on my way to Fall Creek. I was questioned as to why I was going "Shane the body will be out and recovery will be done by the time you could even get there, so why are you going"? This statement bothers me to this day and my answer was simple but my reply was "We have a ranger (Brent Measles) who has been sitting with that little girl's body for several hours during the investigation and waiting on the medical examiner and he needs our love and support.

It was early in the morning when I arrived at the park inn where I found the manager Jacob Young and ranger Brent Measles and all I could do is hug Brent and thank him for his service. I knew he was physically and mentally whipped but we sat on a bench out in front of the Inn for a few hours and I let them both just talk. There was still a mountain of investigation to go and worries about the brokenhearted father but I can never appreciate all of the rangers and responders on this case enough for their service.

This is a perfect example of "why God made a Ranger"! Well done they are good and faithful servants!

FALL CREEK FALLS GHOST

Late one night I received a call from park manager Jim Hall at Fall Creek that they had a potential suicide jumper at one of the overlooks at the scenic loop just past the big falls. The night ranger, Cara Alexander was closing up the scenic loop when she spotted a vehicle at one of the overlooks. As she walked out to the cliff she yelled for a response. After several minutes of no visitor contact, ranger Alexander returned to the vehicle and found a dog in the vehicle, and under further plain view inspection she found a note on the dash that read the fact that the man stated he had jumped over the edge.

Ranger Alexander began to contact other rangers and supervisors and a search was about to begin. After Jim Hall got there the car was unlocked so they retrieved the note for further inspection. It read who he was and that he couldn't deal with life anymore and he said we could find his body at the bottom of the cliff (and he even drew an arrow). He also stated who his next of kin was and the phone number where he could be contacted along with the location of all of his insurance papers that could be found. He also left the number of a girl we should call to come to pick up his dog and where the food for the canine could be found.

Jim called the brother and his brother agreed that he more than likely jumped since he had attempted it a few times in the near past, especially since he had refused to take his medicine. At this time it was already dark but rangers and rescue personnel decided to rappel off the cliff to see if they could find his body but also in hopes that he may still be alive clinging onto a rock or tree. This decision was a tough and dangerous but selfless act by the rangers, but they were hoping to find him only injured. In this area, there is no safe or nearby way to get to the bottom of the cliff.

As the night grew longer Jim gave me a call to let me know they did not find his body anywhere at the bottom and they were attempting to ascend back out of the gorge, by now it was around 2:00 a.m. Jim and I agreed we didn't think he could have survived the 165-foot fall and wandered off into the gorge but with nobody we had to assume anything. Jim asked if I could assist at daylight with a plan and resources, but since the weather was stormy and raining I knew getting a helicopter would not be an option from the Tennessee highway patrol but there was a good chance we could get a UAV or drone from Maury County EMA so I set the wheels in motion and decided to meet Jim at first daylight.

My colleague Tommy Henley with Maury County would be on his way that morning so I decided to go on up and get an early start on the planning process. As I arrived I noticed a ranger vehicle parked at the gate entrance to the scenic loop so I pulled up and found that Cara Alexander (who was the night closing ranger) stayed up all night at the gate in case the man somehow made it back to his truck and attempted to leave. I was so proud that she had dedicated so much time to the search and taken such quick actions when she first spotted the vehicle. I told her I was not brave enough to stay there all night by myself! About this time park manager Jim Hall pulled up to our two vehicles at the gate and I asked to read the note to see if there was anything that seemed odd to me.

I was having a little trouble reading the note since the sun was just attempting to peek over the trees and darkness was still present. As I stood beside Jim's truck straining to read the note I had this odd feeling there was something out in the darkness and I stopped reading to scan the horizon behind the gate after a few seconds out of the darkness of the woods I spotted something or someone walking out of the woods about 20 feet beyond the closed gate. As I tried to focus my eyes and convince my mind what I was seeing my eyes made contact with a man looking at me but walking hurriedly across the road and headed back into the woods. Without hesitation, my body involuntarily took off and jumped the gate and ran into the woods as the man was beginning to run from me!

This was almost an out-of-body experience since we were 3 or 4 miles from his vehicle in the opposite direction he told us he was headed to jump but I knew of nothing else to do but make verbal contact for him to stop, hope he was not armed or wanting to harm to me! I knew I had to make contact with him before he got too far into the woods or we would have a mess on our hands with a ground search but for who, was this our man? I made the decision I was going to tackle him and put a stop to whatever was going on but in the back of my mind I heard my inner self tell me but "What if this is just a park visitor out for a jog"!!

As he was about to enter the brush he would not stop at my command so I grabbed him with a bear hug to stop him in his tracks! His eyes were glassed over and it took him a few minutes when I got him back to Jim's truck to get enough information from him that this was our guy. He had not jumped and wandered around in the woods all night and what luck that was it on our part that he came out of the woods right in front of us!

We transported him to a hotel room to talk with him and call his brother to come get him. As we began to ask about his night he said he just roamed through the woods all night and it is unbelievable that he didn't walk off a bluff at night. We probed him a little further about if he went to the edge to jump and he never would address the issue. His brother came to get him and other family members took his vehicle after the district attorney was okay with our investigation.

Once they left Jim and I went to the park restaurant to eat lunch when an old friend and co-worker Mike Gaines (who I hadn't seen in several years) came over to our table to say hi.

After a few minutes of hello's, Mike said he went to the scenic drive the day before and he walked out to one of the points he said a man was standing on the edge so close that he looked like he was about to jump off the edge. Mike said he asked the man if he was okay and he just turned to Mike with a blank stare and just walked back toward his vehicle. I told Mike our story and that he probably interrupted the man and subsequently probably saved his life.

After our meal, I spent a few hours with Jim patrolling the park and discussing what a major search we would have had on our hands if we hadn't found him at daybreak! As I exited Jim's vehicle he sarcastically gave me the Jim Hall smile and said "After all of our hard work all night I guess you are going to take credit for finding him"! I looked back at my friend and said with a smirk, " Of course"! I sure miss my friend!

FALL CREEK FALLS

Unfortunately, there are too many suicides in our world, and state parks are not immune to this topic. As you may know by now I have worked many suicides in many different forms and it is an interest of mine not to the point of interest but why and perhaps how to prevent it. I have worked directly or indirectly with park rangers across the state and with many agencies with my bloodhounds on over 75 suicides.

A few that haunt me are two we had at Fall Creek where I worked with my mentor Jim Hall. Jim asked me to assist with the investigation of a woman who jumped from the top of the overlook at Fall Creek. The lady had stayed at the park the night before so Jim and the investigators started there and I began to work on her background. It seemed she had been suffering from bipolar personality issues that I got from interviewing her therapist but due to Dr. client and HIPPA laws, I could only dig so far.

There was a note in the room but it only rambled on the life issues that were too much but did not give an absolute answer to the suicide. There was also a large amount of empty alcohol bottles of vodka found in the room. Sometime late in the evening the lady made her way to the overlook and jumped. Another life was lost before we could get them the help they needed.

The second one at Fall Creek was a very tough case of a young man who was from a prominent family but had struggled with his ability to be a college student and so drifted from small job to job. For some unknown pressures in life, this young man found himself like so many in America every minute to take their own life and he chose Fall Creek.

One thing I have learned from many suicides is that they may leave evidence that their body is in a certain area for someone to find or they don't want to damage their personal belongings. On this date, this young man walked to the overlook from the parking lot and took off his shoes, watch, wallet, and eyeglasses, and then just jumped to his death. This behavior could be for others to know something is odd and to look for a person below or is it just from our upbringing not to get our clothes dirty or not to break our glasses?

After working with the local sheriff investigators and then removing his body I did the toughest job of my career that I have done many times, telling the family. The parents lived in a nearby county so it was not a long commute so I made that long walk to the door and rang the doorbell. I would not want to put this pressure on anyone but it unfortunately is the next step on the incident and has to be done to let the family begin the grieving process. On this late evening, the door was answered by an older gentleman, and after a few introductions, I knew this was the father of my subject.

There is no easy way to break this news and you never know how the families will take the news and on this date, it was not good. The father began to become very agitated and screamed at me that this could not be true and then he broke down to tell me the problems he and his son shared over the years for his son's future. He seemed to experience many different types of emotion even to the point of physical altercation but that is just an example of the emotions during this time.

After an hour or so the man had come to grips with the information and was somewhat now calmed down. As I said I do not wish this on anyone and we all need to keep an eye on each other to recognize the warning sign of suicide.

FALL CREEK FALLS DROWNING

In mid-June of 2016, the assistant manager at Fall Creek Falls Andy Wright contacted me and told me he had a report of a missing man around the cascades at the nature center. It was believed he might have drowned but no one from his family or any other visitors saw him go in the water. I responded to assist where I could, and rangers were already searching the cane creek drainage. Interpretive specialist Stuart Carroll had been snorkeling in the water below the cascades and above cane creek falls but he had no contact with the man.

When I arrived the first issue we had to tackle was a communication barrier because the family did not speak English. There was one family member who spoke a little broken English but not enough to get a good account of his whereabouts. The family was playing and swimming at the cascades at the nature center just above the swinging bridge and the last time they saw him he was walking downstream towards the swinging bridge when he disappeared around the corner. I contacted the "Watch Point" at the Tennessee Emergency Management Agency in Nashville to see if they could get me a clergyman who could speak Spanish and it took a few minutes but they found one with Metro police in Nashville.

As rangers were searching for the man Andy and I began to retrace his steps in attempts to come up with a few guesses of where he may be. One, he could have slipped and fallen anywhere from the point last seen, second he may have gone swimming around the swinging bridge and drowned, he also could have gotten out on the trail and was lost, and lastly, he could have walked to the cane creek overlook falls and possibly fallen off the falls and drown in the plunge pool.

As the day was growing to evening rangers had cleared the area above the falls and ranger Matt Brown and seasonal rangers Kayley Kempton and Gillian Roberts were searching the drainage. Gillian went in from Fall Creek trail and worked her way towards Cane Creek where she met Matt and Kayley had searched some of the side trails. At this point we felt he may have gone over the falls and drowned so I called Matt Majors with Tennessee Wildlife Resources Agency and asked if he could assist with his underwater UAV.

Matt showed up around dark that evening and several of the rangers and I helped to transport his equipment down the treacherous "cable trail". Once we got down the trail we carried all of the equipment to the plunge pool of cane creek falls and Matt deployed his rover. The rover is an unmanned machine that is handled by a remote and it will scan the water and the bottom with a side scan sonar and camera. Matt being the professional that he is combed the pool all night long as we sat there staring at the screen in hopes to find our missing man but unfortunately, we found nothing so we decided to call it off for the night. We were all exhausted from a very long night and it was early into the morning as we began one of the toughest climbs up the cable trail. The trail is almost straight up and is tough at best, but it was miserable carrying equipment and I was carrying a 50-pound Honda generator.

As we reached the top of the trail I looked at Andy and said with my most sincere voice "Folks you just witnessed my last trip up the cable trail"! We all decided to get some rest and try again in the morning. We laid out a plan and agreed to meet again in the morning.

We met that morning at the nature center and once again tried to come up with an area to search. We decided to open the area back up at the swinging bridge to the public because we felt he may have floated downstream. As we were working to get adequate resources to search downstream we had a report at the cascades that his body floated up from behind a rock. He had slipped as he walked downstream and hit his head and fell into the water, and drowned with no witnesses.

FALL CREEK FALLS CAMPOUT CARRYOUT

Late one evening I received a phone call from area park manager Steve Pardue that the manager from Fall Creek needed a few dozen rangers to assist the next morning at daylight with a carryout. A woman had taken approximately 26 kids on a hike from the cable trail and would come up the Fall Creek drainage which is a very hard hike for the best of hikers. Not even is this a challenge for anyone the lady did not take into account the time of day which was late in the evening before they even started their trek!

A call came into the rangers of the group being overdue so a search was conducted by rangers Robin Bayless and Stuart Carroll. After a long evening in the arduous drainage, the group was found but by this time it was around 11:00 p.m., and as the rangers evaluated the group it was discovered that the adult leading the group had a broken ankle so it would take several dozen responders and hours to get her out of the rocky creek. After several minutes of discussion by rangers who had done this carry out hundreds of times and what made it more challenging were the 25 or so scared-to-death kids! It was determined they did not have enough people to get her out safely both for her and the responders so, the idea was to have a "campout"!

Rangers built a fire in the creek bed and other park staff brought some blankets and pillows in an attempt to make the kids and patients as comfortable as possible for the long night. My job was to assemble a large group of rangers (at midnight) to be at the park at first light to go in for the carryout so, as I made all of the calls waking rangers up they did what they all do so well, they said "I will be there Chief"! Rangers all across the state interrupted a good night of sleep, threw their pack in the truck, and began to descend on Fall Creek. I loaded up our rescue trailer and headed toward Fall Creek as I had done so many times!

I was there by 3:00 a.m. at the Fall Creek overlook and thought I would try to get an hour or two of sleep but as soon as I dosed off rangers began to arrive so it was time to get up! I met with Jim Hall and we put a plan together to send in a group of rangers and rescue squad members with a rescue basket to package the injured woman and a second group of rangers to assist the kids. Around 5:30 a.m. we held a briefing of the task at hand and first light all the responders set off with their marching orders.

For many, you may have hiked down to the base of Fall Creek which is a pretty challenging hike with rock steps and rails but what most folks have not done is hike the drainage which is a hike from hell! There are boulders the size of cars you must climb over with your fingernails and toenails because they are slick from water and slime then there is the large number of spruce trees that have come down from ice and wind storms that add another challenge to cross over!

As responders arrived, rangers Ray Cutcher and Sturt Carroll who had been with them all night with no sleep began the process of packaging the woman for the long carryout. Other rangers and responders began walking the kids out but as the day and the carryout loomed on it was obvious we did not have enough people to do the job. I left the command area and met the teams along the creek bank and took several kids with me so others could go assist with the carryout. In attempts to put it into perspective, a carryout is tough on flat ground for responders but we had a few miles over the boulders and trees so it takes dozens of people to not only carry but others have to run ahead of the obstacles so the patient can be passed to them and the process just keeps going all the way out!

As I was bringing a group out I decided to take a shortcut to the top that Ray had shown me years ago to save a little time rather than coming up the trail to the falls. I never would have thought the walk with the kids would be so hard because they did not like my pace but also one of them was scared to death when any bug or fly would land on them so my patients were pushed to the limits! We all kept pushing toward the top and it was a relief to get them to the top.

We all rushed to the bottom to assist and relieve the group that had done the brunt of the work all the way and there is no greater joy when you make the summit! As we made our way to the top some of the responders were "cramping up" but the rest of us kept up our pace until the job was done, then we all fell to the ground!

We all took a long break then took turns thanking each other for the help and began our long drives to our homes. You had to have known the manager Jim Hall who was a particle joker but also a penny pincher with his budget so as I was crossing the dam in the park I heard a radio from the inn asking "Jim, who should we charge all of the cookies to we brought to the rescue and without skipping a beat Jim quickly, the Chief rangers office"! All I could do is grin and shake my head and say "he got me again" but I was wrong!

The next week I was re-organizing my rescue trailer as I did after every rescue when I realized I had used my backboard for the carryout so I called Jim and said "Make sure you get my backboard back from the ambulance service" which should not have been hard since it was bright yellow with bold black permanent marker on it saying "Ranger Program Property". A few weeks later I was there at the park for the folk festival and I went to the park office to meet with Jom but also I went to the area where they kept all of their rescue equipment and when I opened the door I spotted my backboard or what I thought was my backboard.

As I inspected the board there were no inscriptions on it so I walked back to Jim's office and said "It looks like the magic marker was removed" Jim just grinned and said, " have no idea what you are talking about"! I knew Jim was a miser when it came to buying equipment for the rangers so I just took it on the chin for my fellow rangers!

** As a follow-up to this rescue I was refueled by a campaign I had started a few years ago after another terrible carry-out by begging anyone who would listen to me that we needed a rescue hoist helicopter for situations like this but it was always a money issue! I barely could replace a backboard much less a hoist but I would keep going to THP and Captain Tommy Hale who had always been a great friend to state parks and spent a lot of time going through the mountain rescue classes.

DROWNING'S ON DUCK RIVER

Even though this has been an exciting and rewarding job it is also full of sadness and heartbreak. Late one afternoon several kids were swinging on a rope swing on the far side of the river just below the boat ramp. One young man attempted to cross the channel wearing long blue jean pants and cowboy boots when the weight of the water and swiftness pulled his body under the surface. I was at our farm cutting trees when I was contacted by Johnny Hobert from the inn and I immediately drove to my office and grabbed our rescue boat.

Ranger Patrick Dwyer and I launched the boat with rescue equipment and traveled to the point last seen. My training and experience have taught me the body is usually right below where he was last seen and we drug the area for several long minutes. It had been about an hour and a half since he went under, so Patrick and I moved the boat downstream into the bend and began our dragging efforts again when Patrick said "I think I have got something"! He began pulling the rope until I spotted the young man's blonde hair appear in the murky Duck River water and at this point, I lunged over the side of the boat to grab his lifeless body!

Even though he was a teenager his water-logged body was more than I could pull over the side so Patrick jumped beside me and we wrestled his body into the boat. We then sped downstream to the waiting ambulance and then struggle with what has always been the hardest part of my job in telling the parents of the young man he was gone.

JULY 4TH DOUBLE DROWNING

I was working the weekend at Tim's Ford state park when I received a call from Brad Halfacre that two men had apparently gone under and swept away on the river adjacent to the picnic area. I responded as well as many of our local rescue squads and fireman along with local TWRA officer Doug Lowery. As I drove to the park I was called by assistant director of Maury County EMA Mark Gandee and he just happened to be driving by the park so he was able to get to the scene and lay eyes on it for me. After his synopsis, I then requested the Maury County swift water dive team to assist us in the recovery.

As I arrived the park was full of emergency workers and vehicles with several rescue boats on the water. One man was wading from the shoal into the water when he found himself too far from the bank and the swift water drew him into the current when a family member jumped into the river in an attempt to save him but the tragedy of the story is that both individuals could not swim nor were wearing life jackets. The horror of the day was the other family members witnessed both men being drawn down the rapids and then their life on earth faded out as the bodies slowly are pulled under in the river.

TWRA officer Doug Lowery was working his boat in the area with a drag while the rescue squad was working the same actions from another boat. Soon one body was found and several minutes went by as we were attempting to get the dive team in the water when another drag boat discovered the second body. Our biggest challenge in the emergency came the family could speak no English so there was an issue to gain good information on the description and age of our swimmers.

This brought a sad end to what is usually a celebration for that family but is always a reminder of our job to be prepared for anything!

DIABETIC DROWNING TAILGATE DROP

It was a very awesome day in my career that was even better than when you get a new vehicle but after many years of trying I was able to get a 4-horse gooseneck trailer. I had just returned from the dealer and before I left the owner sat me down to talk about gooseneck trailer advantages and issues. Guy Wallace was the owner of " Guy Wallace Trailer Sales and Service" and he told me since I had only pulled bumper hitch horse trailers in my career I should take my tailgate off when I got home so I don't damage it. He went on to explain that many people will forget about the neck and they will close the tailgate and put a dent in the tailgate when they pull off.

When I returned to my office I backed the trailer into the barn and began slowly going through all of the procedures to unhook the trailer. I dropped the tailgate, scotched the trailer wheels, unlatched the neck, unhooked the safety chains, and began to raise the trailer off of the ball, and within a few minutes, I was successful.

Before I could do anything else I heard the hotel clerk trying to get in touch with the ranger but he did not answer. The clerk called again and I could tell there was stress in her voice so I radioed the clerk and asked what she had. She stated the lifeguards needed help because they had a woman in the water having a diabetic seizure and they cod not control her and were afraid she was going to drown.

I immediately jumped out of the truck, made sure the trailer was hooked, and then did the sin that Guy warned me about; in a panic, I slammed the tailgate shut and took off with my sirens blaring. As I took off I heard the thump and as I looked in the rearview mirror I saw my tailgate flying in the air.

I made it to the pool to help rescue the woman and get her into the ambulance and get her packaged. For several months I drove my truck without a tailgate, mainly because mine was in the shape of a perfect letter V!

DEREK LEUKING SEARCH
IN THE GREAT SMOKIE MOUNTAINS

On March 16th, 2012, I was contacted by Chief Ranger of the GSMNP, Steve Kloester about me bringing a group of rangers to assist in the search for Derek Leuking, a 24-year-old recent college graduate from a bible college in Knoxville and was living and working in that city. Co-workers contacted Derek's family when he didn't show up for work (which was very out of character for him) and they rushed to the area and began their search for Derek.

They were able to find a reservation on his computer for a micro-hotel in Cherokee, North Carolina and they quickly made their way to the spot but only found a bible on the bed and a bottle of liquor on the floor, which raises some concerns possible he was upset or concerned about something! Just by chance, they found his abandoned vehicle in the GSMNP at the New Found Gap parking lot, so they thought he may have just gone for a hike.

The family made their way into the vehicle and found a note that said he was" gone into the wilderness and don't come to try to follow me or find me because you won't. Oddly enough NPS rangers found a receipt for over $1000 of survival gear in the car but he did not take any of the equipment with him. To a trained investigator this points to a fake search or a potential suicide but his dad dint believes his son killed himself, however, he had noticed some changes in his life lately that were concerning.

Despite the oddness of the case, Chief Kloester initiated a search of about 60 search professionals that searched dozens of trails and rugged off-trail areas for clues. My team which was made of Anthony Jones, Jacob Ingram, and Mark Matzkiw was sent towards the North Carolina side of New Found Gap in some of the most rugged terrain I had been in for some time! After hours of searching in a tremendous downpour of rain, our area was completed and no teams found any clues.

What also made this search tough for the NPS staff was the fact that another abandoned vehicle had been found in a parking lot close to the Sugarlands visitor center, so we had to send part of our search teams to that area in search of Michael Giovanni. After a week of searching the park system called off both searches in the park, however, six months later a skull and backpack were found within a mile of the parking lot and it was determined to be that of Giovanni.

As to the writing of this story in late 2022, Derek has never been found in the park or the rest of the world.

DICKSON COUNTY VEHICULAR HOMICIDE

One Sunday afternoon I received a call from ranger Megan Dunn requesting my advice and the use of my k-9 to find a potential suspect who had crossed the center line on Highway 70 in front of Montgomery Bell state park and struck a smaller vehicle in which a 16-year-old girl was killed and the driver was seriously injured. The ranger stated the driver of the vehicle that crossed the center line was missing and had fled into the woods on park property. I told her I would be responding in a few minutes and it would take me approximately an hour to get on scene.

When I was approaching Columbia I contacted Ranger Dunn by phone to make sure the subject had not been found and I did not want to continue to run emergency traffic through the town if not needed. When I talked with her she said he had not been found but an officer on the scene said I wouldn't be any help with the dog so there was no need for me to keep coming....well if you know me very well this only fueled my desire to get there and catch the guy under their nose! I continued my travel west and with most manhunts, I thought I would give THP aviation a call since they work a lot of events on Sunday just to see if there was a chance they were in the air. When Lt. Lund told me he was in the air but was flying to a murder scene I knew he was out but he said

Sgt. Lee Russell had just dropped him off in Nashville and was headed back to Carrol County so we got him diverted to the park and I had him to start searching the area.

As I continued I was given information on the suspected driver from his driver's license and I asked Sgt. Russell to fly a direct line from the point of crash to the suspect's house which was only a few miles away. I was positive with the terrain and size/age of the suspect and the possibility of him being injured he more than likely had not covered very much ground and was hiding or possibly dead himself! As I arrived on the scene there were serval county and state officers on the scene and I noticed a k-9 officer on the highway approaching me and stated he had the scene and was working his dog looking for the suspect. Well again I was not very happy so I told the officer I promise you he is not out here on the highway after two hours!

I was more than ever now determined to find this suspect especially if he was still in our state park, so I had Lee fly the route again and I drove down the road a few hundred yards to the first house and went to ask permission from the land owner to drive back in there field to the wood line that backed up to park property and as expected they were more than happy to drive back in attempts to find him. As I used my experience and the line of travel I thought he would have taken I drove to the furthest back corner of their field. I was in constant communication with THP pilot and park manager Pat Wright as he was with Captain Travis Plotzer patrolling the campground since it was not far over the hill from where the suspect direction was anticipated. I told him I would be checking the woods with my k-9 in an attempt to pick up his scent and would keep him posted.

I exited my vehicle and went around to harness my bloodhound and as I was hooking her lead up she was already interested in some type of scent and immediately drug me into the woods and by the hard drive and excitement I expected her to very soon pick up our back guys trail when all of the sudden she drug me into a downed tree where I spotted a man lying in the branches and as so many times before my bloodhound drug me right up to the subject! I immediately challenged the suspect at gunpoint and soon decided he was too lethargic or injured to run. I immediately became concerned that the suspect may be injured but before I could get to my truck and retrieve my medical kit I was afraid the distance would allow him to run so without back up I was not sure what to do!

I have had a great working relationship with THP Aviation and we all have a great respect for each other's talent so when I radioed THP 71 Sgt. Russell instructed him to fly to the scene and find my truck in the backfield and land beside it and hold the cover on the suspect while I searched him for weapons and also attended to any injuries he may have.

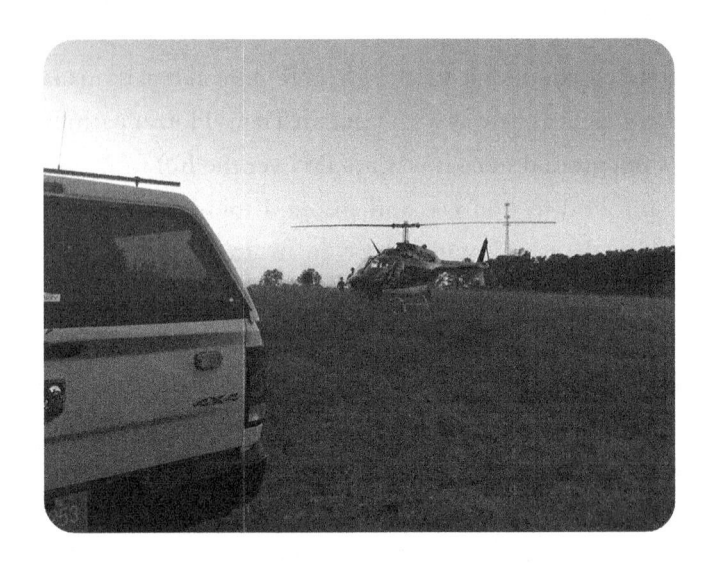

Once I broke the radio silence all of the local officers were trying to find where I was located but since I had Lee I just let them squirm a little while I basked in my find! Also about this time I radioed park manager Pat Wright and let him know I had the suspect in custody and he stated; "you weren't even on scene and found him in 10 minutes" and I quickly told him, "6 MINUTES"! After I searched the suspect I was trying to determine if his lethargic state was from a possible head injury or if it seemed more obvious he was intoxicated on something as he barely could answer any questions and kept dosing off. I checked his pulse and blood pressure and did a quick head-to-toe survey of any injuries and except for a few scratches he seemed to be okay, however, I was very concerned with what seemed to be a swollen cherry-red tongue and thought he must have bitten it in the accident. It was later told to me by the THP investigator he had been drinking a cherry slushy!!!

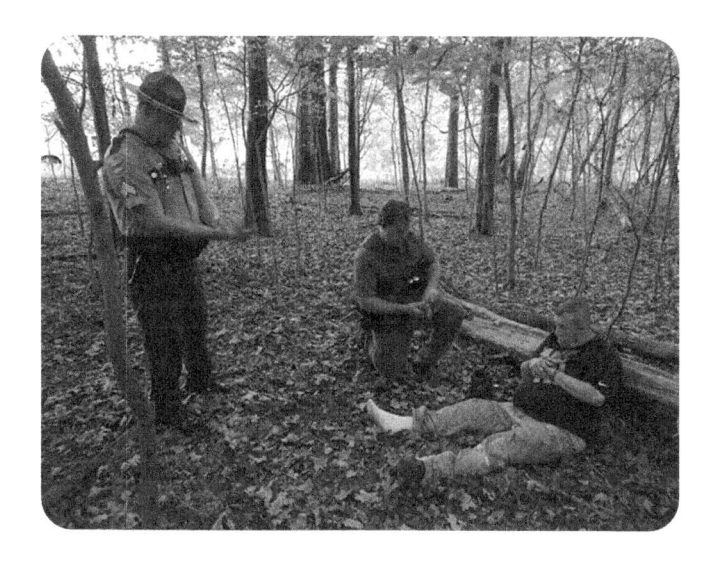

After several attempts to ask the man why he was there and trying to understand his mumbling he kept passing out and we just decided to load him in the ambulance. As of this writing, he has not gone to court but I hope to testify in his hearing and convict him of vehicular homicide!

Update: After several delays due to Covid, Sgt. Lee Russell, Sgt. Denny Mitchell, and myself testified in the court hearing and helped him receive a 55 year sentence for the family.

This was my last case and last time I worked with Sgt. Lee Russell.

CUMMINS FALLS DOUBLE DROWNING

On June 17, 2014, I received that heartbreaking call I have gotten so many times over the years, that not only one kid has drowned but 2! At the time Cummins Falls was in its infancy as a park but the summer was in full swing. On this day a non-profit group from Nashville had brought 39 kids from a summer program to the park and like all visitors they ventured down to the falls and eventually the swimming hole.

Several young men jumped into the 9–13-foot depth swimming area and unfortunately many could not swim the group's leaders and other guests jumped into the pool in an attempt to rescue them. Several of the boys were pulled to safety but 2, 13-year old's did not surface. Information was relayed to the park office immediately and the park began a frantic search for the boys and began to implement the local resources to assist in the rescue.

The local rescue squad responded, and divers were put into the water but they were not successful in finding the boys. The park manager and my closest rescue partner over the years Ray Cutcher called me and informed me of the situation. I have been on dozens of rescues with Ray, and he is the calmest and laid-back person I know.... but this day he was very concerned about the situation. There was no success in finding the two young men with all the resources, the families were beginning to arrive as well as the media. Ray had to only say a few words, 'Shane get me some help"!

I knew from his tone he had too much on him and I began doing what I did best, rallying rangers and resources for a response. I immediately began a text blast to our search and rescue team members of the situation and we needed them to respond at first light the next morning. My second move was to contact another rock star in this type of emergency, Matt Majors with the Tennessee Wildlife Resources agency which oversees water safety and their UAV program (which is a remote underwater sonar and camera search device). Matt agreed to be at the park as early as he could even though I was requesting at daylight because I wanted to give our best efforts in now what was a recovery mode.

One of the areas I had gotten such great help in situations like these was the ability to re-hab or feed the many personnel I was bringing to the park. I made a call to Fall Creek Falls state park manager Jim Hall that I would need almost 90 "hiker ham" sandwiches for the next day, which meant a request to the restaurant manager, Zonda Holloway, who has always been there for us. Her team arrived at the park the next morning before dawn to begin cooking for our team members.

My job was then to begin our rescue response by requesting my seasonal Mark Matzkiw to hook up the rescue trailer and I began to hook up our mobile command trailer for the early morning response. During the evening I was in constant communication with my boss Mike Carlton and area manager Steve Pardue along with dozens of rangers. I completed our search plan and relayed it to Ray and set a goal to recover these two young men for the families by 8:00 a.m.

As with so many responses in my career, we left early in the morning with our caravan of rescue resources. Because our response of rangers would be limited since it was in the middle of the summer, I asked members of the Maury County emergency management agency to assist me with incident command especially in the matter of accountability (which is keeping up with every rescue member who came to help to ensure they all return safely, and no one is left behind). My partners from Maury EMA were Tommy Henley and Mark Gandee and they were diligent in their jobs!

As rangers began arriving we sent several down to the swimming pool to begin a new search, seasonal Mark Matzkiw began setting up a rope hoist system to get equipment down to the recovery area. We had several rangers waiting when Captain Majors arrived, and they hustled as rangers always do to unload his equipment and then make the arduous task to get the heavy equipment to the site. Ranger Jeremy Vaden grabbed two armloads of equipment and took off like a goat down the mountainside.

Local rescue and law enforcement members were also beginning to arrive as we were putting our plan together as now an operation. One of my dearest professionals with the Tennessee highway patrol is Captain R.C. Christian and this day just like many before he provided me with two troopers to man the gate so our rangers would be free to search. As we were beginning to get Matt and his equipment into the pool the family were beginning to show up. This situation is always the hardest to manage to ensure you are doing your job to find the bodies for the family but to also provide the appropriate sympathy. On this day we were blessed to have a chaplain with Jackson County to assist us with the family.

All rescue professionals are taught to do everything in their power to keep the family as comfortable as possible in a designated area and discourage them from assisting so the professional teams can do their job, however on this day the mom and the dad were dead set on being there for their babies, so we decided to get them as close as possible so they could see the operation but not hinder the work.

At 7:21 a.m. I heard ranger Jeremy Vaden call over the radio the bitter-sweet communication that we needed a "green air splint", so if you recall from the earlier chapter this term is to let all of our staff know a body has been recovered. As we began to document and send recovery equipment down ranger Vaden communicated again back to me at the command center at 7:39 a second "green air splint". As I stated this is a bittersweet call but we know the search is over and the recovery can begin and then the grieving process for the family.

The rangers and other personnel began the process to bring both the young men out of the gorge to awaiting ambulances and we did our best to pray and comfort the families at this point. This is always the hardest part of the job, to find the appropriate words to comfort them but continue the job to get your people and equipment out safely. At this time, I also had a call from Jim Hall who was en route with 85 "hiker ham" sandwiches to feed our folks but when I asked Mark Gandee how many workers did we have on the check-in list he stated "88". I told Jim to come to the park and as luck would have 3 members of the local rescue squad had to leave so when he arrived everyone was rewarded with a Fall Creek special!

We concluded with our debrief and thanks to Matt and his professionalism and sent our teams home even though it was a tough outcome, this is why God made a ranger!

CUMBERLAND TRAIL NORTH CHICK LOST COUPLE

In early April of 2007, I received a call from ranger Daniel Basham of the Cumberland Trail that they had two teenagers that had gone hiking on the trail very nearly dark. They were not prepared hikers as they lived in a nearby neighborhood and were more out on a date away from their parents. The parents had contacted Ranger Basham and they did what the C.T. ranger did best most of their lives, hit the trail to find the lost!

After a long and exhaustive search of several miles of trail to the loop rangers couldn't locate the teens so, that is when I get the call. "Bash" gave me all of the details and with every search I look at the weather and age of the lost person and that determines our "search urgency"! It was early spring but the weather was seasonal warm and the teens were young and strong so we decided not to risk the safety of any other rescue personnel in the treacherous mountains. I decided since they went in there as a couple, they would get a chance to hug all night!

I made a call to the emergency agency for my friend Brad Lund with THP to see if he could fly it the next morning but I had talked to him earlier in the day and knew he was scheduled to assist Maury county sheriff's department with their annual Mule Day but maybe he could give me a few hours. As I called the agency a supervisor told me the pilot was out of town and I became pretty furious and called him directly in the best Brad Lund professionalism he said " I have to be in Columbia at 11:00 but I can give you a few hours.

Due to many incidents in this area, Brad and I already had our landing zone close to the park so I agreed to meet him at the LZ at 8:00 a.m. I arose early and drove to meet Brad and help the C.T. rangers with the day's search. This is a very steep and dangerous trail where one wrong step can lead to a severe injury so we were prepared for anything but very concerned since the kids were not found on the trail and did not return home. Brad landed in our designed bank parking lot landing zone and took off for the trail in search of our lost hikers.

The trail was still under construction and not yet connected to other areas of the trail but the trail is inside a 7000-acre natural area so we knew they could be lost deep in the wilderness. The trail climbs from the two entrances to the top of the gorge above the North Chickamauga Creek for several miles but eventually drops back into the creek gorge. I am not positive of the altitude from the tree tops to the creek but it has got to be a few thousand feet in elevation so when Brad topped the trees he made no hesitation to drop down into the gorge almost giving me a heart attack but you cants see from that height so we began our search. Unfortunately, the canopy is very dense in this area and this time of year adds many leaves so trying to spot them on the trail or off the trail would be almost impossible so, Brad decided our best bet would be to fly the creek drainage hoping they may have made it to the creek safely.

We had only flown the creek gorge for a few minutes we Brad said, " I got 'em"! They were cold and huddled together as expected but fortunately, the sun was helping to warm the rock so we were glad they were in good shape. Brad flew over them so we could get a thumbs up from them and then he asked if I had extra water in my bag and he lowered down to pitch the two bottles of water. I said, "Wouldn't be better for me to do it since you are flying"? In Brad Lund's cool demeanor, he said, "This ain't my first rodeo, give me the water"!

We were able to relay the coordinates of the two kids to ranger Basham and Brad flew me back to the truck where we both made our way back to Columbia for Mule Day, of course, he beat me by 4 hours!

BURGESS FALLS HIGH ANGLE RESCUE

In mid-March of 2021, we were conducting a high-angle rope rescue class with rangers from all across the state taught by our close partners from Hamilton county cave and the cliff team at Fall Creek Falls. This class was a long-standing tradition from the early days of Mountain Rescue taught by Bobby Harbin. As the team was wrapping up lunch close to the big falls a call came to me that a man and woman were hiking in a closed area of Burgess Falls fell. The information relayed to me was the man had fallen from an unknown height but was severely injured and was in a very dangerous area beside the flooded water.

Even though the manager said he thought they could handle the rescue with the local response but could use a few rangers for the carry-out. After conversations with the teams and instructors at Fall Creek, I decided to send everyone, which was around 50 responders. I knew it would take away from the learning objectives of the class but the students would never be able to get the experience they were going to experience on this real response!

We all loaded up and packed into vehicles and raced to Burgess Falls which was only about 25 minutes away. I was on the phone back and forth with the park manager and area manager on the situation when the patient reports were coming in the man was very severely hurt. He had fallen about 20 feet while attempting to climb the falls and the area was compromised from flooding. The conflicting reports coming in did not sound very good and the area manager requested me to get a rescue helicopter from the Tennessee Highway Patrol aviation unit.

I made communication with the helicopter pilot and waited while he worked to get a rescue team ready for a response. As I got to the scene teams from the local area were already assessing the victim who had multiple fractures including an open fracture that required a tourniquet to stop the bleeding. Our rangers and Hamilton County worked with the locals to formulate a plan to use a rope rescue scenario. Luckily we also had members of the Appalachian Mountain Rescue team with us which included Dr. Bill Campbell who is an emergency room trauma doctor and one of our lead paramedics Jeremy Vaden so we could not have had a better medical team with the victim.

There was a lot of confusion on the best rescue route but it was all dependent on the location which was on a rock only a few feet away from the roaring flooded water and the only route out was straight you the 65-foot cliff face. With still so much uncertainty on the ability to get the man out I told THP to come onto the scene. THP had partnered up a few years before with the Nashville fire department to have their paramedics and trained helicopter hoist technicians to respond with THP.

The team finally had the patient packaged to begin the hoist when the haul system anchored by rocks gave away and the patient was only barely off the ground so no injury to him was caused. What was adding to the already arduous scene was that the patient weighed approximately 300 pounds which stretched all of the equipment. About this time the helicopter arrived and was surveying the scene from above to see if they could make the rescue from the air.

Unfortunately, some of the teams were not very happy with me calling a helicopter but in situations like this, it was a tough life-saving decision to make. The teams on the scene felt they could get the victim out and the helicopter could dislodge rocks down on the teams and patient. Several workers discussed the rescue and it was determined to continue with the rope team so the helicopter landed in an open area beside the park.

It took another hour and a half but the teams had the man out and brought him to the top to place in the waiting ambulance to transport to another helicopter from Vanderbilt Life Flight for transport to the trauma center. As myself and assistant chief J.R. Tinch inspected the patient we could tell he had an open femur fracture and potential internal injuries. We assisted the teams to get him across the lot to the waiting helicopter.

As expected, my THP team was too happy with me that they didn't get the chance to hoist and sometimes politics can get in the way of emergencies when agencies struggle to get along for the greater good of the patient. As the pilot and good friend were leaving, he let me know about the future response when he said, "If you need us call us but, if you call us, need us"!

BURGESS FALLS GOAT MAN

A call came in one day from Jason Chadwell that had just graduated from the police academy and was stationed at Burgess Falls he was frantic about a visitor who approached him and said a 13-year-old boy had fallen from the top of the waterfall. I instructed him to get as much information as he could and that I would be there as quickly as possible, so I left Nashville and made as many calls to emergency workers with rope and dive skills to meet us there!

When I arrived, rescue workers were already searching in the water for the young man and I began to re-interview the witness of exactly what he saw and remembered. He told me he visited the park every morning to drink coffee and explore and watch the goats that would climb on the cliffs. On this day he stated he was walking down the creek when he witnessed a 13-year-old boy go over the falls. He struggled to give me a good description and clothing but I continued my interview I was just not getting a good feeling about the situation of the witness, so I asked him to take me to exactly where he was standing when he witnessed the fall.

As we got to the point and showed me everything I surveyed the area and assumed that he could not even see the top of the falls from where was standing and soon I was beginning to smell a rat! I had just graduated from the FBI National

Academy and I thrived on interview and interrogation so I was anxious to give it a shot. I decided to jump in with both feet and told the man there was no way he could see the falls and I believe he was not being truthful with me about the whole situation! A normal person who had witnessed the terrible accident would become outraged when challenged about their telling the truth, but he just stared at the ground.

As I gained further information on the man he told me he was a roofer and he just really enjoyed the park and that is why he came every day but I knew from working on several roofs you try to get the work done as early in the morning as you can before it gets too hot and we were in the middle of the summer! I then began to challenge his story of working for a roofing company and also I was very curious about the goats because we weren't in Colorado and we don't have mountain goats! When he began to stumble on his story I knew he was not telling the truth.

I began another tactic to confront him vocally that I believed he was living and he made the story up just to get attention and as I awaited again his demeanor I got nothing but a stare at the ground. I decided to continue the "bad cop" routine by putting pressure on him that he would be responsible for anyone of the rescue workers if they got hurt looking for no one, but still no reaction. I decided since I didn't have another experienced interrogator with me I would try to switch roles and now be the empathetic "good cop" and see what would happen!

BRAD LUND

Brad Lund and I have had a tremendous relationship that is twofold. It first began with our two state agencies' long relationship for search and rescue but also as I became in demand as a k-9 officer in Tennessee.

I met Brad around 2002 when I had put together a rope high-angle rescue class at Fall Creek Falls with TSP and THP special ops. Brad graciously agreed to bring the Hughey up for us to begin the first rappelling operations from the helicopter in state parks. I say this because Brad had the forethought of how important the aviation section was going to be able to assist us in search and rescue but also his desire to TRAIN us!

Our relationship began soon after that when I was being requested by so many police and sheriff's departments for my k-9 for many non-violent and then violent criminals where Brad became very familiar with my k-9 ability but he always made sure to keep me in his view during a search not just to help to find the subject but for MY SAFETY!

In 2004, Parker Ray Elliott killed his ex-wife, and 17-year-old daughter, and shot his son 7 times. I spent most of the first night clearing buildings in and around the home but Brad also was in the air with me at every step. During the next several days we spent many hours in the Maury and

Lawrence County line looking for Parker Ray after his vehicle was found in the area of Military Road. After 4 days of searching some witnesses' saw a man fitting his description run into the woods. I was called to the area with my bloodhound and began a hot track, as Brad heard the radio communications he quickly flew to the area and spotted me but also spotted our killer, Brad strategically moved the aircraft to the opposite side of the tree so Elliott would have his back to me and his eyes on the helicopter which allowed me to rush to our killer and take him by surprise at gunpoint so no one got hurt. Elliott still had the weapon in his jump bag but because of the stealth of the aircraft he had no idea I was on him and he could not make any defense moves. I got all the credit for the find but Brad was the real hero that day! Certainly, that afternoon Brad Lund kept me from getting killed and he also kept me from having to use deadly force by just maneuvering his aircraft! I became his biggest advocate and he was my hero after that day!

<In the years since Brad and I have worked on dozens and dozens of criminal searches, me on the ground with the dog and he in the air with night vision, FLIR, cameras, and all sorts of equipment but he has always made sure I was safe on the ground!

<In 2005 he responded to Montgomery Bell to assist me with a missing person in the park where we had found her car. We suspected foul play or potential suicide. Brad left a mission and picked me up on the ball field and we began flying the lake at the park when he spotted the body of the lady submerged 10 feet below the surface. He was able to bring

closure to that case which would have taken us a few days until the body would have floated up.

<In 2009 TSP began opening more areas of our park system called the Cumberland Trail. One early April day we had two young people who did not come out of the woods after their hike. I called Brad late that night and he said "he had to work a big traffic control event in Maury County the next morning but he could give me 2 maybe 3 hours". He picked me up and flew the steep gorge canyon of Single Mountain and he immediately spotted the two down in the creek drainage. He gave them two thumbs up, we called into rangers their location and then he flew down into the gorge and dropped two bottles of water to them while they waited for the rangers to get to their location. He dropped me off and made it back to Maury County to work the big event there. Later that evening he and I were reunited in the woods of Maury County to look for a missing man who unfortunately took his life. All in a day's work for Brad Lund!

<in 2011, we were beginning to ramp up our rope and helicopter joint training with THP when I was getting word of a new park in Jackson County (Cummins Falls). After seeing it in person the hundreds of people hanging off the cliffs I knew I would have my hands full with accidents and rescues! I asked Brad when our rope training was finished could we fly over to the park and look at the possibility of doing a hoist out of the gorge. We flew over and down in the gorge and he gave the thumbs up for the ability. It didn't take long for us to call him on a drowning subject where Brad was frustrated he couldn't fly done in the gorge and load the patient in the

small aircraft. My viewpoint was he could land down in there in the small aircraft, so late one evening after a storm ran visitors off I received a photo via text from Lt. Lund of his helicopter sitting on the sand bar! A few weeks later he picked me up and we practiced several loads and go pick-offs if we had to load a patient in an emergency down in the gorge.

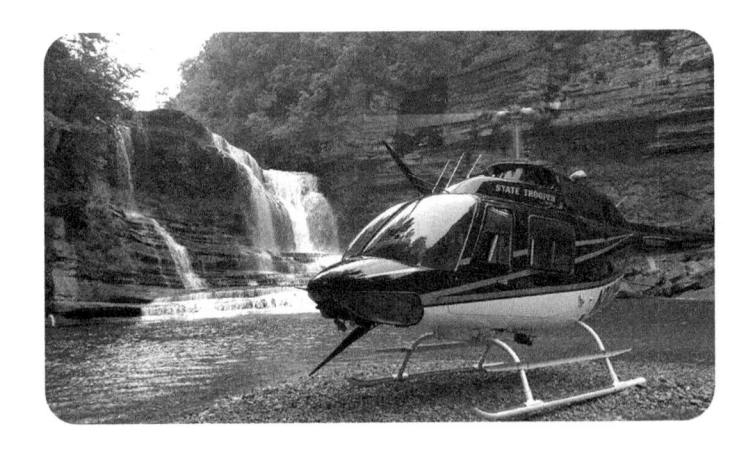

< In 2018, we had one of the calmest 4th of July weekends on record…..until I received a call from Brad on July the 5th that said we had one of the worse emergencies he had ever seen at Cummins Falls, He informed me of the flash flood where waters rose 4 feet in 4 minutes and so many people were trapped on rocks in the middle of the river. When I asked if he was going to go back to Nashville to get the Hughey he said "These people will die in 5 minutes if I don't do anything" Then I lost his call. His next actions are the bravest thing I have ever witnessed in the state of Tennessee in which he flew down and loaded a park ranger with life jackets and flew over and dropped them down to the family

stuck on the rock (soon after that one of the family members was swept away and because they had on the life jacket they floated right to a ranger in the water). Brad then without regard to his own life lowered the skids of the aircraft down into the water and picked up each family member one by one and delivered them safely to the parking lot. Not only did Brad save their lives off the rock I was there when their daughter who was swept away was reunited with them and they knew she was alive!!!

Unfortunately, the mother of the man on the rock was swept away so Brad kept searching for her but to no luck. After the family was safe he noticed several individuals safe but stranded high on an island. He flew back to Nashville, jumped in the Hughey, and came back to hoist 9 people off the island. The next morning he picked me up in Nashville and we flew all day in search of the missing mother until we spotted her lifeless body. Not only did he do one of the biggest rescues in the state's history he also brought closure to the family by bringing the mother and grandmother of the family on the rock by finding and bringing her body back.

In the following days, I attended her funeral and I was a little apprehensive about how the dad would welcome me. As I told him how sorry I was for his loss he smiled and said, "Today is a great day, my mom lived a great life and we could be here with 5 caskets"! Those caskets were not there only because of the ability, training, and preparation of Brad Lund and his commitment to his fellow man!

Even after we brought her body back, Brad has not finished learning. He and I flew upstream until we could find where the rain had settled in one concentrated area to cause that much flood water. I came back that day a much wiser and richer human but also I knew I had witnessed the greatness that I may never see again, from my hero!

In the last several years Brad and I have teamed up on numerous trainings where we teach search and rescue and manhunt operations from the ground and air perspective. He has assisted me dozens of times when I teach at the police academy for each basic police school, we have taught for several ranger and rescue teams, and last year we teamed up to teach for THPs in service. He is very dedicated to teaching others to help save time and money for the state.

Unfortunately, I don't have a good number of how many times I have called for his assistance but it ranks in the hundreds. He gets requested by every state, city, state, and federal agency around and he never lets us down. I know personally his family takes a back seat to us way too many times but he knows when we need him he is there for advice, protection, and tactics. He has always got our 6!

If there is a more dedicated Tennessean out there we would be hard-pressed to be beat Brad, he is a true Tennessee hero!

BRAD LAVIES,
THE SEARCH THAT CHANGED MY LIFE

On March 28, 1993, a young boy from Alabama was hiking along the rainbow falls trail with his brother Chris and his mom and dad Nancy and Randy (along with a friend of the family when Brad became separated from the family as he ventured up ahead of the family. This was the first time the family had spent hiking the Rainbow Falls trail and as the members were ascending the trail to the falls Brad began skipping switchbacks to shorten the hike as he raced ahead of his family.

Because he was sprinting up in front of them, they did not notice he had gotten off the trail and was missing until they arrived at the falls. Brad's dad began a frantic search for his son on the way down the mountain and when he could not find Brad, he got hold of the park service.

Rangers Benny Sledge, Dave Panabaker, and Steve Kloester began organizing a search for the young Lavies later that evening, however, Brad was nowhere to be found. After several hours of searching the duo began the establishment of a search plan and calling all rangers and staff into the park the next day to assist with the search. The next day (Tuesday) the search was expanded to areas of the trail where Brad may have become lost off the trail and the lead rangers began to plan for an extended search they reached out to the Tennessee Emergency Agency area coordinator Bob Swabe for assistance in resources from Tennessee.

Tennessee state park rangers had begun classes with TEMA on man tracking and search operations management through Bob and Richard Taylor, so Bob was quick to reach out to TSP and Chief Ranger Ed Schoenberger. Ed and I quickly put together a group of rangers and made our first of many trips to the "Norma Dan" motel in Pigeon Forge. TSP rangers mustered up quickly to get their rooms late into the evening of Tuesday and met at first light on Wednesday to receive our briefing from rangers at the visitor's center. From there were transported back through Gatlinburg and then to the Rainbow Falls parking lot where we began our hike up to our search segment.

I was assigned to a group that would search the rugged area off-trail towards the drainage from the falls while another group of rangers headed up by Stuart Carrol and Randy Hedgepath hiked and searched areas where the trail from Rainbow Falls intersected with the Mt. LeConte trail in hopes they would find Brad or other hikers who may have seen him on the trail. Their job was to camp and stay at the intersection for 3 days.

As the days kept moving with no signs of Brad the search grew bigger in scale and more assets were brought in such as helicopters from the Army National Guard as well as k-9 teams such as Richard Taylor (who would become one of my great teachers, mentors, and friends for the next 30 years!

Richard had the first k-9 certified in Tennessee to search standards named Osh. Search teams were sent downhill from the trail thinking Brad may have become lost and tried to find his way towards Gatlinburg since you could see the lights at night from this area while others were sent to a higher rugged area towards the falls.

On Saturday, April 3, 1993, our team was sent to a very rugged drainage that would lead almost up to the falls, an area that had been searched by another team but due to the dangerous steep terrain, vegetation, and issue that Brad was wearing a camouflage poncho team would research this area. Around 12;30 p.m. a call came over the radio that the team beside us found his body at the bottom of a ledge about one-third of a mile from the Rainbow Falls trail at an altitude of about 4,800 feet.

It was determined that Brad died from massive head trauma after slipping and falling from an 80–100-foot rock ledge. This search included over 300 search professionals both paid and volunteers. The reason this search changed my life was the fact that every day we came out of the woods it would break our hearts to see Brad's mom and dad in the parking lot and we had no information to give them about the whereabouts of their son.

I began my quest to be the best search and rescue ranger I could be through equipment, training, and preparation. I began taking more classes from Bob and Richard about search tactics and management as well as specialization areas which would eventually turn me into a bloodhound k-9 handler for the next 30 years under the watchful eye of Bob and Richard who were both outstanding k-9 handlers as well. I also began to lay the groundwork for my version of the national program "Hug a Tree', which was developed by a mom after her son had been lost it teaches kids ideas to keep them safe if they become lost as well as things kids and parents can do to help plan if their child is lost. Over the next 30 years, I was able to facilitate this program to over 1000 groups and approximately 100.000 people, including every child who went to Marshall County schools!

In 2019 I made contact with Brad's mom and dad who live in Alabama but also own a home just west of Gatlinburg. They so graciously opened their home up to me and shared their story of that week. We both told our versions and shed tears together, but they did find comfort that his death was a chance for me to educate and teach thousands whom I will never know but will always believe I saved someone's life from Brad's story. When I asked Randy and Nancy what advice they would give they said, "Keep a close eye on your kids".

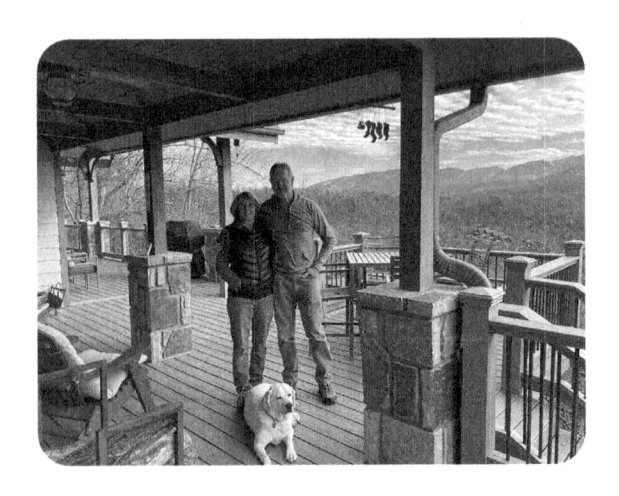

In early 2000 I was called to Foster Falls to assist with a missing person but she was not lost in the woods but missing from the parking lot! A group of 4 came to the park to rock climb at the popular site but one of the individuals did not want to go to the bottom, so she decided to stay at the top to sunbathe and read a good book.

As we questioned the individuals it was found they were from Atlanta, Georgia and she had no other means of transportation and knew no one else in the area. When asked if she would get in the car with a stranger they said sternly "No" She is very paranoid with other people, so I took off with my bloodhound while other rangers worked the bluff areas but we all were concerned about an abduction.

We had tried all our friends and family members in Atlanta but could not locate her anywhere, so we kept pushing ourselves into the woods to find her. At the end of the day when we reached back at the parking lot with no sign of her we began to re-group and make a decision on our next search tactic for the following day when I decided to try the mother again and inform her of her missing daughter.

As I gave my best detailed information of what had happened and what we were doing as an agency to find her the mom finally chuckled and said, "I doubt you will ever find her up there because she is here in her room asleep!" I asked the mom to wake her and let me talk to her and get the story from her when I learned a big lesson in the search arena because there are always two sides to every story!

The girl had been very upset to be there in the first place and certainly did not want to go rock climbing but got so mad waiting on them that she just walked up to a car in the parking lot that had Atlanta tags and asked for a ride with a total stranger! I was proud of our job but disappointed that the other folks were not 100% truthful.

ARROW SUICIDE

One afternoon I was contacted by rangers at Long Hunter state park about a potential suicide. Rangers were checking the parking lot before closing up the area and could see a note in the vehicle that the subject was going to commit suicide. I was out of town and could not make it with my bloodhound but we were able to get Nashville metro in on the search with boots on the ground and aviation assets. After several hours the search was suspended and they would try to interview friends and family to find further clues.

I contacted the best k-9 handler I know Richard Taylor to bring his dog and cadaver experience along with ranger Bridgette Loftgren from Hiwassee/Ocoee state park to work with him. The day before I had used a k-9 group I had never worked with but used them on a reference from an associate I respected and they had told me the dog showed he was not in the park, but they didn't know we had him on a security camera going onto the hiking trail and never coming out (never used that group again)!

As we arrived, rangers began the search and we found the subject in the woods 30 yards off of the trail dead from a single gunshot wound. During searches, we now look at lost person behavior, and from my experience with so many suicide cases most (not all) people do not want their bodies laid out in the woods for animals to attack even though they are dead so that is usually why they leave notes or other clues.

My partner and other search expert Tommy Henley went with me to help support the incident and we knew our subject was a heavy smoker since his ashtray was full and dozens of butts were in the floorboard. As we made our way to the body we found on the trail an arrow pointing to the body with his brand of cigarette butt in the middle of the arrow, a clue that he was trying to tell us where his body could be found. (This has taught us in the future to always look for clues)!

A NIGHTMARE AT STANDING STONE

One day I received a call from the park manager Chris Cole, and he was inquiring about a massive sinkhole that was on forestry land. He knew I had worked a homicide case in the area a few years before in which we suspected the estranged husband had killed his former wife and potentially dumped her in a sinkhole Chris had received a request from the sheriff's department on another similar homicide where it was thought from some information another man had dumped a girl in a hole.

The manager asked if I could remember where the sinkhole was located, so I gave him my best directions but also warned him that there was no way to see down in the hole since it was several hundred feet in depth but the biggest warning I gave was that you had to be tied into an anchor because the entrance was like a funnel, big at the top but step to a smaller opening but it was extremely dangerous.

The manager explained that to the group with another ranger and a couple of deputies so as they were making their way to the sinkhole one of the young new deputies took off running to the area when he tried to slide down to take a look into the dark hole he slid right down the hill of the funnel and disappeared into the darkness of the crevice of over 200 foot.

I was in West Tennessee when he called me back frantic I had a bad suspicion about what had happened. I felt so bad for Chris and all I could do was get him some technical rope teams on the way as it would take a lot of rope and technical rope experts and a lot of time to get his body out. Unfortunately, as expected the young eager deputy was dead and there was no body of a woman down in the hole either.

The sad thing for me was as the young deputy had just graduated from the academy and I knew from teaching there that he had talked to me about being a ranger. A very sad day for the department and his family.

MY LAST SEARCH AS CHIEF (AND IT WAS OUR BIGGEST)

It was a very cold evening on February 3, 2021, when ranger Jeremy Vaden called me concerning a vehicle that was still in the parking lot after closing hours and it was dark. The vehicle was from Ohio and there was visibly hiking equipment and a backpack in the vehicle which seemed to confirm that the occupant or persons in the vehicle more than likely came to the park to hike but no one could seem to find them. Jeremy told me that ranger Neal Weatherley had gone down the trail towards the waterfall and the park manager went downstream in case he missed the trail coming back to the top. Jeremy was just giving me a heads-up on the situation and believed they would find him soon since not very few people get lost at the park.

In the search world, we look at several factors to determine the level of emergency such as: age, is the person by themselves, gear, and preparation, and the biggest one is always WEATHER! My concern was the weather because at 6:00 p.m. it was 23 degrees and even though it is a hiking park you are surrounded by water over half of the trip and then the main attraction is the waterfall! The rangers and manager knew the urgency as well and they were clearing all of the trails as quickly as they could in hopes of bringing the search to a quiet ending!

By now you know my job is to bring the masses to the incident, but I was in a holding pattern until they cleared the trails like a good scout, I texted my partner Lt. Lund with THP just to give him the heads up. After about an hour the rangers came out of the gorge, but they had not found anything or anyone. Ranger Vaden began to dig into the investigative side of the house by running the tag and doing good work to locate the vehicles owner's dad (Robert J. Qusai II) who lived in Ohio and confirmed that his son (Robert J. Qusai III) had left from the dad's house headed to Tennessee to hike some waterfalls. This investigative work is crucial as it is another confirming piece of the puzzle telling us it is more than likely a real missing person in the park however, there is always the possibility that the person caught a ride or went to eat dinner with someone, but the dad said he did not know anyone in Tennessee.

As the night grew longer with no hiker to be found I hated to request a helicopter so late that night, but the weather was just too much of a factor especially if had fallen into the water! Jeremy had continued his efforts on the investigative side by getting the cell phone number and first calling it but there was no answer. He then worked with Jackson County and Putnam County to "ping" his phone, but one showed his phone was over 4 miles and the other showed it to be a mile away, so Jeremy traveled to the area but found only an open empty field. Jeremy was in constant communication with me so when he drew up empty with phone pings, I called one of our partners at TBI.

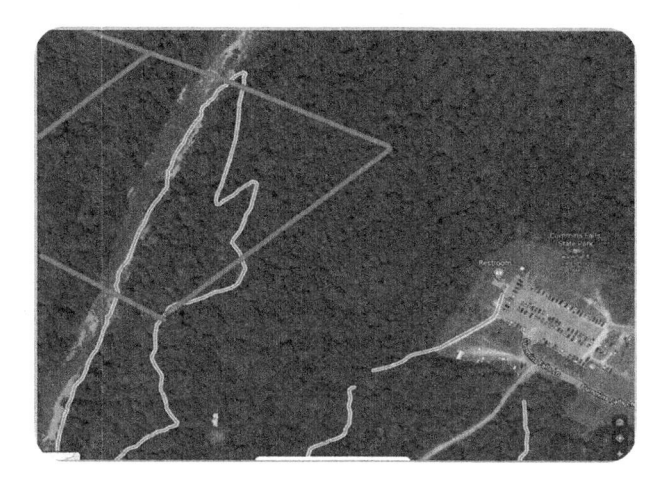

Andy Vallee was the lead cell phone forensic technician with TBI and had become a close partner in situations like these and he was always very helpful. He took all of the information and even shared it with his counterpart with the FBI and they confirmed a much closer ping with the phone and sent me a triangulation of where it was showing the phone to be and that was down in the confluence of the river where the trail crossed the creek, so we sent a crew to that area in search of any clues but found nothing.

By this time, it was around 11:00 p.m. and I was leaving my house with my bloodhound and Brad was headed to the hangar in Nashville. Even though I was concerned about the weather I was confident that Brad would find him before I ever even reached the park with his new FLIR (Forward Looking InfraRed). THP had recently received a brand-new

Bell 469 helicopter that could match the muscle of the Huey but was much quieter and stealthy, but it had a new state-of-the-art FLR. I had recently flown with Brad on a training mission to look for wild hogs in one of our parks and as we were flying you could see raccoons in a tree from over 2000 feet in the air.

As I got close to the park, I could see Brad and Captain Steve Lowery in the air and I couldn't believe that had not found him yet. The FLR picks up heat from anything but Brad also had a very sophisticated camera so you could tell a human from a deer I was positive with the cold weather Brad would spot him in the gorge where he may have missed the trail coming from the creek when it got dark on him. As I got to the park, I still felt comfortable that Brad would find him but I was growing concerned since he had not been spotted at this point, so park manager Cutcher and all of the rangers began to lay out a plan. We knew at this point where his phone was last pinged in a triangulation at the creek and trail confluence and from all information, we had from Andy with TBI the phone was still on so a few of the rangers went to the bottom to see if we could see or hear the phone but once again no luck!

Brad searched the entire gorge and adjoining landowners to the park for several hours, but he could not come up with anything so as he left back for Nashville I began to become very concerned as to wear our hiker may be or if he was injured. As Jeremy was digging into his life from social media and the father, we had a little more eye opener of who our missing hiker was and where he may have gone that day in the park. Ranger Ashley Clark Woolbright hiked the trails on the top and others went to the campground across from the main entrance and knocked on several campers' doors to see if he had maybe made his way to them and found warmth, but no one had seen our hiker.

As we began to dig deeper into our subject, we found information that he was a lawyer but from a general Google search we found information that he was about to be "disbarred" by the Ohio supreme court and upon our further inventory of his vehicle we found some prescribed medication that unfortunately led our mind to the possibility of suicide, but we kept positive this was not the case. Before I got my bloodhound out, I made a "Ready Ops" text to our rangers across the state to assist us in the morning.

At this point I got my bloodhound out "Swabe" to see if we could trail our subject since, we now had an article of clothing from the car, so I chose our strong man ranger Neal Weatherley to go with me into the gorge since Swabe is a high energy driving dog and there are a lot of bluffs in the park! We trailed him for a while on the trails then she led us to the creek where I expected her to lead us up to the waterfall, but she kept us in a circle for several minutes in the creek bottom and across the creek. After several minutes we just could not find our way to a direction so I lead her upstream to see if she would pick up his scent but there was no alert by Swabe so we began to work downstream to see if that would show more scent but after working downstream for quite a way, we could not find his scent.

Neal and I made the arduous climb straight up the cliff to see if maybe we could find his scent on top in case, he became lost in the night and tried to walk back to the parking lot but still no alert from Swabe!

As we made our way back to the office Jeremy and ranger Leigh (like a sleigh) were working with a locksmith in attempts to gain access to his trunk to see if any items in there would lead us to his actions. Jeremy also had begun a look at his tablet and emails along with correspondence with people and Facebook friends so we began attempts to contact them to see if they had any idea where he might be especially in the "ROW" (rest of the world) which is a search investigation theory that he may not even be in the park. To make the situation more of an investigation turn Jeremy found a very variety of illegal drugs in his trunk which now made us think he possibly could have overdosed out in the woods. Our investigation continued with all the evidence we had but we also had to put together a search plan for the rangers who were coming in an hour or so.

We knew it was a long shot but we visited a private campground that is located at the from entrance of the park and knocked on every camper to make sure he did not take cover there to keep warm but there was no sign of Bob.

Our plan was to thoroughly cover the gorge with rangers both upstream and further downstream, but we also wanted to take a look at several small waterfalls that were formed by small drainages from the top. Several of these waterfalls were in a very hazardous spot and seemed that we may have found him in one of those drainages possibly hurt from a fall but as the day grew longer, we still had no luck finding out the missing hiker. I will never be able to express to the citizens of Tennessee and their friends and family how proud I am of our state park rangers and their work to locate our missing hiker. We knew the gorge posed a very serious possibility of injury or death to him but also to those rangers and volunteers looking for him. That is what we call "rangering up"!

After rangers and other agencies hit the trails and gorge, we continued our investigation and our report with the family. His dad had told us he had made two stops on his way to the park from Ohio, the bank and gas station but he also told us he had a few texts from his son; one being a photo from the river crossing (so we had a last known point) and he had received a message that he had lost his sunglasses and was trying to find them. We were sure if he had been lost in the park or wandered off park property, he would eventually find his way to a house or road and make it back to his vehicle but also if he had an accident, we were sure we would find him.

The next awesome resource we used came in the form of UAV's or drones from a group called "Storm Point" who would from that point be a great friend to us! They flew the entire gorge, waterfall, trails, and the rest of the park. They flew around 14 hours on the first day and approximately 36 missions looking at every nook and cranny in the gorge. We had been testing and using drones from several agencies and my great friend from TEMA, Lewis Friedman had been keeping me updated on this storm-point bunch and their professionalism. I will never be able to thank them enough for what they did during those first few operational periods and the relationship that I continue to have with them today. They dissected the waterfall from top to bottom and all points from there to the plunge pool looking for any clues of our missing hiker. I was concerned he may have tried to climb out of the bottom when it got dark and maybe fell and became lodged in a rock crevice or tree, so I asked them to begin checking the bluff walls from the waterfall for any sign.

Even though Brad had given me so much time the night before, I called and asked if he could come back and fly the river drainage to clear the water. Brad in his usual professional manner agreed and flew low covering the park from the falls and about 17 miles downstream his message to me was that the water was so clear and low in most places he just did not believe he was in the water succumb from a drowning.

At this point in the second operational period, our rangers from across the state were beginning to arrive along with many local volunteer rescue personnel so we paired them up in groups to begin a second phase of man tracking for clues and checking the entire trail system along with several small water falls in the gorge. We also began transporting several rangers down to the water to assist in kayaks to look for any sign of our hiker.

We had over 100 searchers out in the field at this point and many of us in the command center began further talking to family and investigating any clues from social media. We found where he had posted a few pictures close to or near the park before he took his hike so we felt again sure he was in the park there was still the idea he may have caught a ride out, but the family believed he knew of no one in Tennessee he would meet up with.

So, after the end of the day or second operational period and debriefing we began to plan for the next day since the area is just too dangerous to search at night, but we left park rangers in the parking lot just in case he walked out. The park staff and my staff began to work on the next operational period planning process. Of course, Jeremy continued with a thorough investigation, and I had several issues on my mind. At this point, we all concluded that more than likely he fell into the plunge pool below the waterfall, so in this case as I have done dozens of times, I contacted my friend with TWRA Matt Majors and request if he could bring his underwater sonar/camera as he has done so many times before. As always, he agreed to meet us there the next day and I was very confident our guy was in the water and just as confident in Matt's ability to find him.

We had another group of rangers coming in the next morning to assist in more areas of the park and drainage, but I kept going back to idea that he may have lost his way in the dark coming back from the waterfall and attempted to climb out of the gorge and fell into a crack. With this in mind I came up with probably my oddest idea to request my friend Brian Krebs with Hamilton County cave and cliff team and ask them to rappel from the top of the gorge and do a grid search to illuminate any small crevices the drones or helicopter may have missed.

I also made a request for air scent dogs from Knoxville to assist in searching areas we didn't have rangers. I doubled checked back with TBI cell phone experts and it was confirmed that his phone was still pinging, and the phone was still on. At this point, we all tried to grab a few hours of rest in what we hoped to be the day we find him.

The next morning, we gave a quick briefing of our plan and sent teams out for another arduous day of searching. Our investigation brought us to a fact that our subject had a few years before left life in the U.S. and wanted to just start a new life in Jamaica, so many of our planning team began to believe he was in the R.O.W. (rest of the world! Jeremey kept going down that rabbit hole when a report came in from a local lady who lived near the park and stated she saw a man the day after he was reported overdue walking down the road. Several of us hit the road and began knocking on doors of houses but after several hours we determined it was a local man who walked the road frequently.

As the day drew on, I was losing hope because Matt was not finding any sign and we he decided to pull out I asked him "How confident was he that our hiker was not in the water?" Matt stated the water was very clear for the camera and a bit low so he could reach almost all the pool and he felt "95% that he was not in the plunge pool." To say the least, I was very let down because I just knew he would find him in the water but there was still that 5% also there was a chance he could be behind the falls so I needed to come up with a plan to search this area, but who could I get for this job since the water had to be around 40 degrees!

I planned with the help of Mike Armistead of the Nashville Fire Department who heads up the Tennessee

"HART" (Helicopter Aquatic Rescue Team) along with Lieutenant Brad Lund who is over the aviation part of the "HART" team. Due to the long and rugged terrain, it would be too hard for rescue swimmers to hike in with dry suits, so we made the plan to hoist them down from the helicopter. Unfortunately, as they arrived in the air the hoist would not work so they had to land and then hike down to the water while Jeremy carried their gear bag. After a few hours, they illuminated the pool and all areas behind the waterfall.

As Matt with TWRA left and the helicopter from THP flew back to Nashville we were so down we had not brought closure for the family but also found ourselves mentally and physically worn out but we had to plan for the next day of searching. At this time the phone stopped pinging and TBI nor FBI had any leads that his bank accounts had been used, so another day of boots on the ground.

Our plan was to hike the gorge further downstream and float rangers down with kayaks 10 miles from the park. We also brought in another group of cadaver k-9s from my dear friend Candy Stooksbury in East Tennessee. By this time the staff felt we had covered almost every inch of the park and I was struggling to keep the energy and spirits up, but I made a request for fresh rangers and they once again rose to the task!

At this point, there comes a time when you wrestle with the fact to scale back due to resources being tired and volunteers returning to their jobs along with officials concerned with the cost of the search. By this time, I had a very good report with the missing hiker's brother, and we spoke every day and then every week as we slowly scaled the search back but we didn't stop. Rangers from the park stayed vigilant every day and we would continue to seek permission to search on private land adjacent to the park.

For the next several months I would continue to call experts on search tactics and body decomposition as well as the rest of the world. I would wake up at night with this search still on my mind and couldn't sleep so I would go to the computer and look at Google Earth to see where I might have missed him. When I would find an area that troubled me, I would just load up and head to the park and spend a few hours eliminating the area of my concern.

I received a call from a local sheriff's department officer about some information he thought might be of interest. On the same day our subject went hiking he had received a call from dispatch about two suspicious people in a convenience store. As the officer arrived, he observed two men leaving the store and enter a vehicle, so he decided to follow it a bit when the vehicle ran a red light and the deputy attempted to pull them over, but they took off at a high rate of speed. The deputy stated their policy does not allow them to engage in a high-speed pursuit for a traffic violation, but he gave me the tag which came ack to an Ohio tag. I ran the tag through dispatch, but it came back "not on file", so it seemed to be a dead end.

I was positive the spring turkey hunters might find him on private land and then hopes the deer hunters in the winter, but all my rangers believed he was not in the park, and I was just spinning my wheels, but with no other information, I kept focused on the park. When we arrived at the yearly anniversary of the search, I got a social media post from a stranger who stated he had noticed a FaceBook sight about the search and what I had done up to this point and that he was an armchair detective from the internet but more importantly he stated that our subjects "All Trail app went live a few days ago". If you are not aware the app allows a person to load their hikes but also friends can see where they have hiked. He also stated that his (our missing hikers) FaceBook sight liked a message on someone's board.

I immediately began to have a panic attack trying to find the sights but at the time my wife and I had our 2 and half year-old twins at the house and they were in a rare form! This excitement did not allow a very good research platform for me, so I immediately called the smartest technology guy I know Clint Derryberry. Clint and I are on the Maury County SAR team, and he also was very instrumental in assisting us at state parks. Clint began the search, and he confirmed what the gentleman told me, our missing hiker had taken 3 hikes post being lost at Cummins in Ohio, Michigan, and Illinois. With this information it was now believed our subject had faked the search but why and how or who helped him?

At this point, I had been talking to his family every few weeks keeping them up to date with everything we were still doing. As Clint began diving further into the technology side, we had to turn our attention to the fact they our missing hiker was not deceased on the park somewhere but how could this be? The next day I received a call from the family and his brother began the conversation like this, "you are not going to believe this, his All Trails went live a few days ago"! As I discussed the new information with the brother, he explained that one of the trails in Michigan was at a state park and the park bordered their grandparents old homeplace and that they had spent much of their childhood roaming the state park. The other hikes where city and county parks that seemed at random, but it was obvious there was something odd.

As Clint continued to work his magic, he discovered that our missing hiker had taken several hikes a few months after the search date at Cummins and several of them were close to his home and even one he (or someone) labeled the hike at a city park "Cummins Falls"! Clint and I continued to scratch our head at all this new technology that seemed to show our guy was in the world taking hikes just as he did in the past like nothing ever happened but how could he do this and still stay under the radar from family and friends.

I began to dive into his past and talk with several of his legal colleagues and even a past girlfriend and several believed that he could have faked the incident and attempted to begin a new life somewhere! Even though the evidence from the technology and friends seem to point that direction and many rangers and search friends believed the same thing I still had a gut feeling he was still on the park. We intensified our investigation on every angle imaginable and I will never be able to thank Clint enough for all his long hours pouring over maps, trails, and social media to learn as much about our missing hiker. Clint knew the names of every family member, where he went to school, what his favorite sports teams where he rooted for, but most importantly Clint made a promise that there was one thing for certain that whenever he was found he would have his college ring on hid hand. Every video and photo he could find Bob was wearing that ring, so if we could find the ring, we could find Bob.

I reached out to and old ranger who had moved up the ranks with the Tennessee Bureau of Investigation, Josh Melton. I explained the issues I was having with the technology and need their help and he bent over backward to make it happen. He put me in touch with an agent who wrote a search warrant for the "All Trails" company. About this time, I called my friend from THP aviation to brainstorm this new technology finds and if he had any wisdom. He told me to talk to Harley with TBI aviation about getting a warrant on a new technology called "Geo-Fencing", which would allow us to find from his cell phone carrier the exact route his cell phone traveled that day. This was a world wind of new technology for me so I relied on my TBI agent Brandon to do the hard work, but he assured me it would be a slow process.

Many believed the new technology had him alive and well, but I still felt obligated to the family to keep looking on the park until further information came about. About this time, I reached back out to my friend Lewis Friedman who was overseeing the drone program at TEMA, and he sent out an email to dozens of state, city, and county agencies drone teams requesting them to assist us in one more big search of the park areas downstream. There were several great agencies that agreed to help us so to lend us assistance on the ground in case something was spotted I asked the Christian based search team of Tennessee to assist. We spent the day searching some of the most rugged and steep terrain along the gorge but after a long day we turned up no new information.

About this same time, I was asked to speak to the MTSU drone program about search and rescue applications and especially what we have done on the Cummins search and many students who had never consider the search application of drones became very interested in this search. Due to the class commitment, they could not be present on the day we had all the drone teams on site, but we set up a date for a few weeks later and they would use what we have done so far and search a new area for us.

When I received a call form Brandon Davenport with TBI I was excited and so he began to tell me what he had learned from the All-Trails company. Unfortunately, they could not give us a definite explanation of how the trails were downloaded post him becoming missing, but they said they believed the information had possibly got stuck out in the cloud and just now downloaded or our man could be out there still hiking! Brandon told me he was still waiting on the search warrant from his cell phone. Our missing hiker was a Google hound which means he stored a ton of information on Google along with photos so we hoped our search warrant from Goggle would bring back some positive information, so we waited.

As winter approached, we began our annual in service training of rangers and even though I believed I had done everything I could I decided to do a briefing with all of our rangers across the state on the search. There was a very positive buy in from many of our rangers as I briefed what we had done but what I was pleased to see many become excited about the SAR program and how they could assist in future searches, especially in the areas of technology. Many of the rangers believed he was in the "ROW" but a few sided with me but I assured them if it was the last thing I ever did I would find him and when I did was retiring, there could never be a search that would top this!

As I awaited any information from TBI I racked my brain on anything else I could do, so I decided to re-visit the vehicle with Ohio tags. I had my local sheriff's department run the tag again and unbelievable it came back this time to an address that was only a few miles from the residence of our missing hiker! Was this just a coincidence or did they come to pick him up? Clint began digging through the social media of the owner of the tags and I began trying to gain information on the tag from local Ohio law enforcement, but they were not very helpful. As I dug further from the family the son of the owner of the vehicle went to school with our missing hiker so now, I believed things were looking like a sham. As we dug deeper the registered owner was shown to have passed away and we could not get in touch with the family and now this was the first time my mind led me to believe he was not on the park!

A few weeks later Brandon contacted me and said he had some pretty good, detailed information from his phone so I rushed it that evening to Clint for him to digest. He called me back that night and said we needed to rally to pour over the ton of information as soon as he cleaned it up a bit. Basically, the information was a 2-minute track of our subjects travels on the day he became missing.

I was blown away at the detailed work Clint had done and as we plowed through the information much of the investigation work, we had done earlier was being confirmed by the tracks. This new technology was so detailed it showed and confirmed what time he left his dad's house in Ohio even to the extent that he backed out of the driveway! He made a few stops, one to a private residence, one to the bank to withdraw money for the trip, a stop to get gas and a direct drive to Tennessee and specifically to Cummins Falls.

Once he arrived at the park, he left his vehicle and walked to the overlook for a few minutes and then took the trail to the water towards the waterfall. Once he arrived to the river, he spent quite a bit of time at the juncture crossing the water back and forth and returning to the opposite side of the river and this location was confirmed from our earlier investigation that he had taken a photo at this point and sent to his dad. This is where the new information got interesting because instead of our hiker heading upstream towards the waterfall, he decided to make the decision to cross back over the river and explore the terrain going straight up out of the gorge. There is no trail in this area and no way to get to the waterfall from this climb so why would he take this route?

As Clint did more work with Google earth, he came to the conclusion that our hiker somehow knew there was a smaller waterfall in the area and he scrambled up the steep wall to find and explore the waterfall. From that point instead of returning to the river and heading to the main falls he continued to climb a few hundred feet up the gorge to the top and skirted the edge of the cliff walking towards the main falls area. When you review the digital track, you can see where he makes his way closer to the falls but would periodically walk to the edge of the cliff top to either gain a view of the waterfall or a view of the gorge below.

His route showed he would return from the edge and continue to work his way towards the falls. The new information not only showed his almost exact tract but also a time stamp every few minutes when all the sudden the track stopped at the edge, but the time stamp and locations continued for 18 hours in approximate the same position.

When I gave the information initially to Clint, he cleaned up the information and was able to confirm that we believed he fell from a certain location at 3:41 p.m. and his phone we believed was 125 foot from the top of the cliff, so the question at hand was the phone still there and could we even find the exact location? I put together a plan with Clint and the park manager Ray Cuthcher and his staff for later in the week to take a new look at the case!

As we arrived that morning and met at the site Clint jumped out of the truck like a giddy schoolboy as he followed behind his GPS. He made a few turns and adjustments and then stuck an orange flag marker into the ground and stated " the phone should be 125 foot below us"! This was the first time I felt he may not be here since we were on the opposite side of the park on private land only 175 feet from the main road. Did he arrange for the Ohio tag car to meet him in this location, hike to this point and throw the phone down the cliff with it still on to keep us searching and believing he was still there or was and his phone 125 feet below us!

Ray is our best rope rescue rangers' hands down, so it was the obvious choice to send him off the edge and even though the location seemed to be far below us he had to search all the way down for any other clues. Ray finally found himself approximate 125 feet down on a shelf, so he stopped to make a thorough search.

One of the best decisions on this day came again from Clint to bring his old metal detector, so we had ranger Lauren Fagin to bring the detector to Ray from the bottom of the gorge. This process took awhile so we skirted the gorge backtracking our missing hikers last known footsteps to a few overlooks and tried to get inside of his head why he was in this area of the park. We returned back to the last known location and waited for any information from Ray.

As we tried to make small talk at the top, we were all on edge awaiting any information from Ray, when the call came in, he had found a cell phone and it was attached to a battery supply which would explain why the phone stayed active for so long! Of course, our plan was hope we find the phone but just as important we hoped there would be some sign of Bob, when Ray came over the radio to inform us, he had found remains of a human body! This now became a crime scene, so I contacted TBI, my administration, and the local coroner. Once the coroner was on site assistant chief J.R. Tinch joined the team in a very rugged area to retrieve the remains. Of course, Clint wanted one more task from Ray and that was to use the metal detector and look for a ring and after a few minutes the call came over describing the ring and we knew our search was over and it was time to bring Bob back home!

As the search team came out of the gorge, I examined the ring with the coroner and TBI agent and the ring had his name inside, so we all felt this was a very positive identification the remains were our missing hiker, but the state medical examiner was not as easily persuaded so we had to take the remains to his office in Nashville.

Even though we did not have 100% identification all the evidence brought us to the reality this was Bob, so I felt I needed to update the family since I had told his brother about the new information and the search were doing that day. It is never easy to inform the family but at least we all had closure.

The next day the medical examiner needed dental records, so I worked with his family to get x-rays and the positive identification was finally made! The next steps were an area I had never been before when the family had questions about how to retrieve his remains and could they be transported, so I leaned to my good friend in Chapel Hill Tommy Howell who owned the local funeral home. He worked out options with the family, so I traveled to the medical examiners office and transported his remains to Tommy where he shipped the cremated remains back home to the family for final closure.

As much experience as I have had searching and running searches this one was a big one and taught us there are no absolutes in the search world. There are many rangers, law enforcement, and volunteers to thank to bring this case to a close but just like every search we do, it is for the families!

ABOUT THE AUTHOR

Shane Petty spent over 33 years with Tennessee state parks with the last 25 as Chief ranger over all emergency training and response. He was also the department's Emergency Services Coordinator for TEMA where helped coordinate all state emergencies for 27 years.

He holds an associate's degree from Columbia state community college, a bachelor's degree from Middle Tennessee State University, and a Masters degree from Bethel University.

He is a graduate of the prestigious FBI National academy and is an adjunct faculty member for the Tennessee Law Enforcement academy for 28 years.

He is on several state committees on search and rescue and is a facilitator and founding member of TSAR (Tracking, Search and Rescue).

He is now retired and married to his loving wife Marla where they live in their log cabin they built on the duck river, spending their time fishing and chasing their 9 grandchildren!

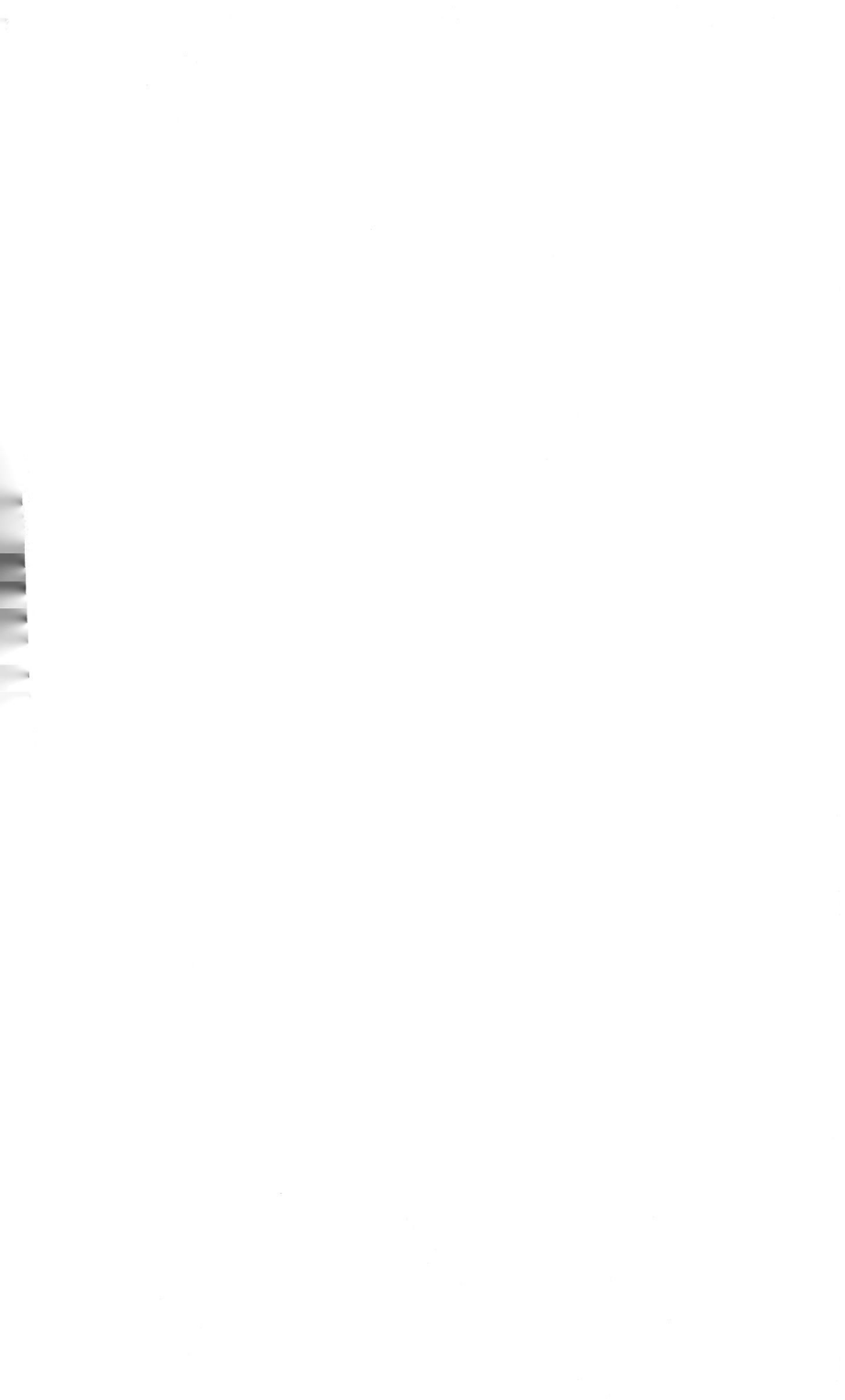

Made in the USA
Columbia, SC
11 July 2025